WE ARE
TITANS!

Contents

PreGame

The first time I gripped a baseball I was three-years old. I remember the smell of the leather, the weight of the ball in my hand and the feeling of the laces against my tiny fingers. I was smitten. Baseball wedged itself in my soul.

As I began learning to play this complex and cruel game, my heroes became the men who made it look so easy, players like Wade Boggs (who ate chicken before every game), Bob Horner (who is only one of seventeen players to hit four home runs in a single game.), Roger "The Rocket" Clemens and Dale Murphy. Baseball was proving to be an impossible challenge for me and I struggled to understand why it appeared to come so naturally to others. As a middle school kid I was inconsistent and during that time, between 12 and 14 years old, I wasn't athletic at all. A short, tubby sixth grader, I remember needing to wear "husky" jeans. I vividly remember being the shortest kid in my seventh-grade class and crying over it because I believed I would never grow. And to make matters worse, I wasn't one of those speedy little kids who took home all the blue ribbons on field day. I was slow… and not a-step-off-the-pace slow. I mean, my time from home to first base could have been measured on the calendar, not on a stopwatch. My arm was also well below par, but I could hit. The best part of my game was hitting, but even so, I was so weak at 14 years old, by the time we transitioned to the 90 foot base path, the thought of hitting a ball with enough gusto to send it flying over the infielders' heads became only a dream. Through all of the failure I concluded the major league icons and college players I idolized must have been ordained by God for the kind of success I could only dream of achieving. Although I believed I would never be a part of the exclusive club reserved for champions and legends, my love of baseball sustained me. For the pure and simple love of it, I worked hard at running, hitting, catching and fielding the baseball and day by day, little by little things got easier. I can't remember when it happened, but I made the connection: the harder I worked at baseball, the better I got at baseball. It may seem obvious, but for me, it was an epiphany. I might not have been able to control the umpires, the opposing players or the weather, but I could control my effort so I vowed to be the hardest worker on the field every single day. Before long I found myself competing with and out-performing even the most talented players. Working to overcome my shortcomings taught me a profound lesson: talent isn't everything. The key to success is consistent, hard work.

I'm not alone in my belief that hard work is the key to achieving maximum personal potential. In his 2008 best seller, *Outliers: The Story of Success*, Malcolm Gladwell examines the factors in achieving excellence and hypothesizes anyone can master a skill with 10000 hours of dedicated practice. It's called the "10000 Hour Rule," a concept he derived from the work of K. Anders Ericsson who studied how people become exceptional. In many cases, especially those involving sports, that study demonstrated hard work has a more profound impact on expert performance than innate ability. (Ericsson, K. Anders, et al. "The Role of Deliberate Practice in the Acquisition of Expert Performance." Psychological Review 1993, Vol. 100. No. 3, pp. 363-406).

Today, as I reflect on the history of Titans Sports Academy, I realize no life lesson has had a greater impact on every facet of our success than the one I learned so long ago. Talent isn't everything. The key to success is consistent hard work. 10,000 hours of practice is a long time, but it's a long time whether you are working hard or not, so why not work hard?

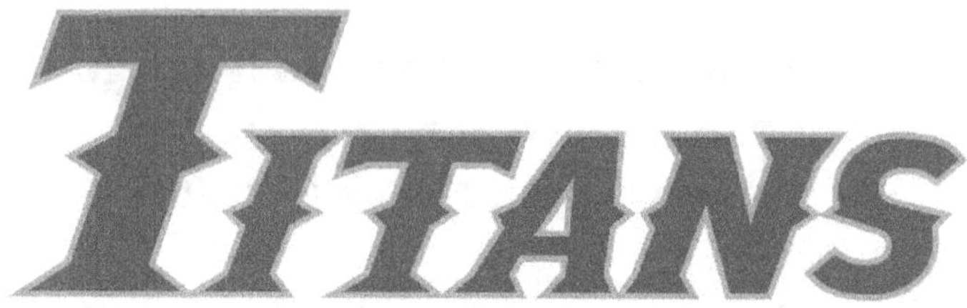

Interested in becoming a Titan player or
want to have a team with us?

Go to TitansNation.net/BeATitan

Inning #1

I loved visiting my grandparents as a kid. They lived in a brick ranch-style house on a hill in Vale, North Carolina with a huge magnolia tree at the very edge of the backyard. One such visit is etched in my mind's eye forever. I was about three or four years old and my grandfather took me outside. He stuck an old, beat-up, wooden bat in my hands, walked about fifteen feet away from me, turned and proceeded to toss me a tattered baseball. Looking back, it's probably lucky I didn't accidentally hit him, but I swung that bat as hard as I could and made solid enough contact to send it sailing over my grandfather's head. My grandmother was out in the yard too, standing twenty or so feet behind my grandfather, and I'll be darned if that ball didn't keep sailing right over my grandmother's head toward the old magnolia tree. I vividly remember the sound of my grandmother's voice as she shouted "Chance! Home run! Run around the bases." That snapshot is my first baseball memory and runs through my mind virtually every day of my life. It represents to me a pure, unadulterated love for the game… no fear of failure, no victory and no defeat… just pure love and joy. It is moments like this one that have shaped me into the person I am today. First my family and then my coaches fostered my love for the game and shaped the principles by which I live my life.

When I was growing up, the travel baseball scene was a bit different than it is today. Back when I played youth baseball there were not the abundance of tournaments, workouts and showcase events to attend on literally every weekend of the year. There were no youth baseball academies and kids didn't take weekly lessons to improve their skills. The only real opportunity for kids to improve their baseball skills 30 years ago was to attend a college camp. Lucky for me, every summer from the time I was ten years old until I graduated from high school, I attended Clemson Baseball Camp.

Clemson Baseball Camp was run by Bill Wilhelm, a legend in college baseball. He was the Head Baseball Coach at Clemson for thirty-six years. When I was a kid, I thought he had been there for at least a hundred years. My first interaction with

Coach Wilhelm came in 1986, during that first summer I ever attended camp. I was in one of the youngest age groups allowed and I remember being driven to Clemson with all my bags packed along with blankets and pillows and bedding. I was going to live in a dorm for a week. I was terrified and incredibly excited all at the same time.

We were housed in Johnstone Hall, an antiquated dormitory which probably should have been condemned, but it wasn't. Johnstone Hall was built in 1954, so in 1986, it was already 32 years old and not air-conditioned. To make matters worse, the dorms were a mile away from the fields and we had to lug our equipment bags as we walked to and from camp each day. Often times we would walk unsupervised. I reminisce about those days, I feel certain someone should have been chaperoning us as we traipsed to and from the field. In today's society the circumstances of my camp days would not stand up to scrutiny, but it was an amazing time. I look back fondly on my time at Clemson during those summers.

During that first summer, I calculated Bill

Wilhelm's age to be somewhere between

one- hundred and one-hundred-fifty years

old. To me he was the greatest thing in the

history of the planet. He could walk on

water and he was going to teach me

everything I needed to know about baseball.

Little did I know that kids in my age group

didn't necessarily get a lot of time with Bill

Wilhelm. That didn't deter me though

because I was excited about the opportunity.

On the very first day after all our parents left, Bill Wilhelm gave a talk which 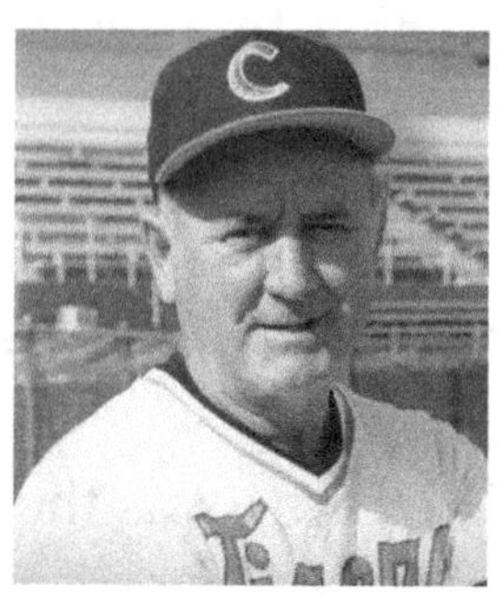 might, to this day, be the most influential speech I have ever heard. It is while writing this book and reflecting that I am able to realize just how much of an impact it had on me. He brought all of us kids in the younger group to sit on the hillside behind Doug Kingsmore Field which was Clemson's Baseball Stadium at the time. He started by telling us he appreciated our taking part in the camp. He told us he was going to teach us the four attributes needed in life for the rest of our days. If that wasn't

foreshadowing, I don't know what was. In

that conversation he laid out the principles

of accountability, responsibility, attitude and

effort. At the time I just thought that they

were words, really big words. Little did I

know that one conversation was probably

going to shape my entire life.

Effort and attitude were the things that he

focused on the most. Effort and attitude took

no athletic ability. This really appealed to

me because at the time I did not think that I

had much athletic ability. Effort did not

require athletic ability. I could make the effort to be the first one to show up to training and be the last one to leave.

Attitude was a bit of a challenge for me because even though I was driven to excel, I had a tough time with losing. I knew, however, that if Coach Wilhelm said we needed positive attitudes and a lot of effort to succeed then that was what I would always aim for. I didn't wait to implement the principles. I started adjusting immediately at the camp.

I got up, ate breakfast and headed straight to the field, where I was always the first one to show up. After a few days, I was able to figure out what drills we would be doing based on the stations that were set up. By the time the coaches finished their pre-camp meeting, I would already be doing drills. At night, I would stay and watch the coaches and camp counsellors clean up. It got dark at around 9:30 to 10 p.m. and most campers my age would be back in their dorms, but not me. I was still out there trying to find something to do, a ball to hit or throw.

Back in those days, only 11 to 17 year-olds

were eligible to attend Clemson Baseball

Camps, and for me it was a summer staple.

While today's youth baseball seasons are

filled with travel teams playing virtually

every weekend with multiple practices

midweek and many weekends scheduled for

travel out of town, I never once had to look

at my schedule or ask my mom if we needed

to talk to my coach about getting some time

off to go to camp. Clemson Baseball Camp

took place in in June and July and by the

time mid-summer rolled around, baseball in

my area had been completed for weeks.

Over the course of my tenure as a Clemson

Baseball Camper, I won the Hustle Award five out of the seven years I attended. I took great pride in out-hustling my peers. I knew I was far from the most talented player on the field, so I had to find an edge. For me it was hustle. I didn't just hustle during drills and games, I hustled between them. When it was time for groups to move from one station to the next, I made it my mission to be first and so I sprinted from one station to the next. Early in those camp weeks, players would try to race me from one station to the next, but I never gave in. One year, my camp group conspired to wear me down by taking turns racing me from station to station. I overheard these conversations and it only served to fuel my desire to out-work everyone. By Wednesday, the other boys lost focus and conceded the hustle title to me. Clemson Baseball Camp provided me seven years of determination, focus positive attitude and what I thought was extraordinary effort and the unintended result of it all: I happened to get better and better at baseball.

During those summers I met people that would have a lasting impact on my entire life. I owe a huge debt of gratitude to Coach

Eddie Hill, who showed me not only what it means to be a great coach, but also great man.

Coach Eddie Hill was the Head Baseball Coach at Rock Hill High School in the early to mid 1990's. He was a lead instructor at Clemson Baseball Camp and he took his job very seriously which made a big impression on me. Having a good time in his words meant, "Getting after it!" Working hard and focusing on the details and nuances is where the average player rose above their own abilities to make themselves something more. I remember wanting to please Coach Hill and wanting his approval. He was kind to me even when I failed. He was tough, but never belittled me. He believed practice was meant to create failure because it is through failure that we learn and grow. *If you wanted to get better at anything, fail more* was his mantra. The way he conducted himself was admirable. No problem too small. He was always available to lend a helping hand.

I was a catcher and Coach Hill was a catcher as well. Naturally I looked up to him with a sort of hero worship as if he was one of the

greatest coaches in the history of the game.

Coach Hill taught me a concept he referred

to as MONA. During camp we would have

defensive specialty sessions where Coach

Hill would talk catching and finer details of

the position. MONA was Coach Hill's

catching philosophy. MONA stands for

mean, ornery, nasty and aggressive. Coach

Hill believed effective catchers are all of

those things. We would take a knee with full

catchers gear on in the summer heat as

Coach Hill explained how a catcher needed

to be mean. A catcher would get foul tips

off their shoulders and ribs, catchers would

take thrown dirt balls from the pitcher off their wrist and forearms and that was expected. If you weren't mean how were you going to battle through that pain of just doing your job?

As an 11 year-old I was not exactly sure what ornery meant. Coach Hill explained it with clarity. He said, "If your dad is watching a football or baseball game and you come in the room and grab the remote and turn the channel, what is his reaction going to be?" Catchers need that same mind set to keep their team on task.

Nasty was my favorite. Coach Hill talked

about how as a catcher if you didn't finish

the game dirty, then what did you do all

day? He explained that a catcher squats

down and is close to the dirt, so just by

proximity you should get dirty. Not to

mention as a catcher

you blocked all balls

thrown from the

pitcher threw to the

plate, even in warm-

ups. If you weren't

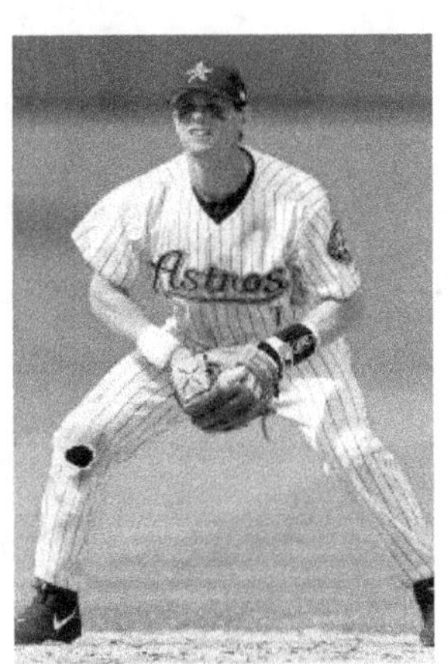

CRAIG BIGGIO HOUSTON
ASTROS

dirty, it probably meant you'd had a bad

day. Coach Hill used Craig Biggio as our

example. During the late 1980's and early

1990's Craig Biggio was a Hall a Fame catcher with the Houston Astros, who later moved to second base. He was the epitome of nasty. His legs would be covered in dirt. He would have pine tar on his jersey and holes in the knees of his pants

As a player I felt like being dirty meant I played hard. When I left the park I wanted to look like Craig Biggio. I believe I probably looked more like Pig-Pen from the Charlie Brown comic series.

Aggressiveness, as Coach Hill explained, was physically being aggressive in throwing to bases in order to back pick runners and control the running game. Aggressiveness was also used in pitch calling. Aggressiveness was not only a physical trait, but also a mental aspect. Aggressiveness could be displayed in just how we took the field. Coach Hill said, "Guys we all know it's hot out here. We all know how easy it is to be tired and feel sorry for ourselves, but when you know all of that and see guys sprinting on the field being aggressive with every action. That stands out!" I owe a lot of my success to as a player and a coach to

MONA.

I was told NO at every stage of my baseball

journey. When I was in junior high school,

coaches told me I would never play in high

school. When I was in high school, coaches

told me I would never play in college. When

I was in college, coaches told me I would

never play professionally. When I began my

professional career, I was told I would never

get in a game. The fact that I was able to

make liars out of all those people is due in

large part to Coach Hill and MONA. You

need to be a little bit mean, a little bit

ornery, a little bit nasty and a little bit

aggressive to turn a no into a yes. Oddly

enough, one of the driving forces behind

everything I have accomplished, both on and

off the field, is having been told no.

When I was I in seventh grade, I played

second base for my junior high school

baseball team. I wasn't very fast, I did not

have a good arm and I couldn't hit. Simply

put, I was not good at baseball. I remember

getting into a game that year and making

three errors. After the game and from that

point forward, the coach stopped talking to

me. He never acknowledged me and I'm

pretty sure he even forgot my name. By

some miracle I made the team again in

eighth grade (barely), but still, I just wasn't

very good at baseball. I was a bench warmer

for most of the season, relegated to mop up

duty, which meant I entered the game when

and if the team was way ahead or far behind.

I did make one great play in that eighth

grade season that sticks out in my head. I

was playing second base in a midseason

game where the everyday second baseman

had gotten hurt. There was one out with a

runner on first base. There was a ground

ball hit up the middle. I watched the bat

make contact with the ball and immediately

broke up the middle. I saw the pitcher reach

to his left and the ball was just out of his

reach. I realized by how hard the ball was hit

I wasn't going to be able to get in front of it.

At the last moment I dove and in a blur of

movement caught the ball and flipped the

ball to the shortstop with my glove never

taking the ball out with my throwing hand. I

can remember laying there, beneath the dust

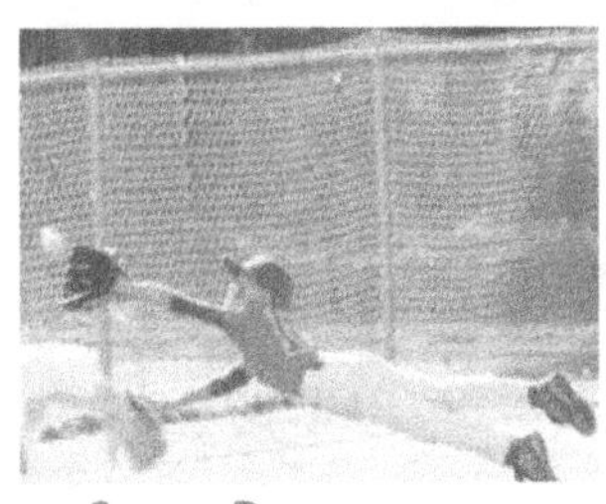

SHANE BARNES DIVING
CATCH 10U

seeing the ball flip

straight up to the

shortstop who was

coming across to cover

second base. He caught the ball, tagged

second base and threw the ball to first base

for the double play. I can remember

thinking… How did that happen? How did I

do that? I was asked the same question in

the locker room by my teammates out of

amazement and disbelief. They asked the

question, waited for the answer and just

shook their heads. It was the first glimpse of

success for me in those awkward middle

school years.

During the summer after eighth grade my

family moved to Clover, a small town in

South Carolina, which was fortunate for me because that's when things started to turn around. Maybe I was a bigger fish in a smaller pond, but suddenly coaches started to notice and appreciate the kind of player I was becoming.

I tried out for my high school varsity baseball team, but ended up getting cut and was relegated to playing junior varsity. Many of the varsity payers told me I was good enough for the varsity squad, but the varsity baseball coach was also the high school football coach. I'd gone out for the football team the previous fall and frankly I didn't make a good first impression. I wasn't fast or strong. I struggled at the game. It became obvious to me Coach didn't particularly like me. In fact, this coach made a habit of favoring the more talented players on the grid iron. If you were an average to below average player, your football experience was very different from the experience of the more talented players, who clearly received preferential treatment. Coaches were more lenient with their talented favorites when they were sore or feeling sick, but the average and below average players were always pushed beyond their limits. The best players were not held to the same standards as the rest of the team. That experience made a lasting impression on me. I promised myself if I ever had the opportunity to coach, the same rules and standards would apply to every player on my entire team. I would ensure equal treatment and a level playing field for all players. To this day, this is probably one of the things I do best. I would even argue that in many instances I hold the better, more talented players to a higher standard. With great talent, comes great responsibility.

Anyway, when I tried out for varsity baseball and got cut, I assumed the Coach was basing his baseball decision on the

impression he had of me from football and I

made it my mission to prove to him that he

made the wrong decision.

I went on and played Junior Varsity that

year. I was the number one pitcher and

caught when I wasn't pitching. I had a great

year. At the end of the JV season, the Coach

brought me up to varsity for the final games.

In the final five games of the varsity season,

I had more hits than all the other varsity

players. I felt vindicated. Without uttering a

single word, I told that Coach he'd made a

mistake. I should have been on the varsity squad all year. In a matter of three years I went from being the least valued to the most valuable player on the team. That Coach told me no. I went from being cut as a freshman to starting every inning of every game from my sophomore year until the day I graduated.

Even though I fought my way to a very good high school career, I was still told no. "Chance, you work really hard. You've got a great attitude, but you're never gonna play college baseball. You're just not good enough." My high school coach did very little to get me on college coaches' radars so, after my senior year I took it upon myself to get a try out at the University of South Carolina at Aiken. USC- Aiken is a Division II school in Aiken, SC.

The coach invited me to try out so I drove down to Aiken, SC and met him at the field house at nine o'clock in the morning. We briefly talked about the program and I went out on the field and played catch with his assistant coach. I got my arm loose by playing some long toss, and made about ten throws to second base. As a catcher you are graded on your "pop time" to second base. This is the time from when the catcher catches a ball until the time the second baseman or shortstop catches the ball at second base. A good college time is 2.0 seconds, pro time would be 1.8 to 1.9 seconds. That day I was a 2.08. The field was already set up for batting practice, so the assistant coach took a bag of balls to the mound and placed them on a bucket behind the L-Screen. I grabbed my bat and took a round of batting practice. I can vaguely remember hitting okay, but nothing special. After approximately 30 minutes of working out on the field, the coach invited me to his

office behind home plate. I sat across from

him as he stared out the glass on to the field

in silence. He simply said that he didn't feel

like I could compete at this level. I

remember sitting in my car to turn on the

ignition to make the drive home. I had been

there for 45 minutes and was leaving with

nothing except a badly bruised ego.

Soon after that disappointing news, I got a

call from Gary Swanson, head coach at St.

Andrews College, an NAIA school in

Laurinburg, North Carolina with an offer to

play on his team. There were sixty-five guys

on the team in the fall. We had so many

guys on the team, we had to fan out from

left field to right field line just so everyone

had enough room to throw to get loose

before practice.

In the very first practice of my freshman

year, I'll never forget, there were nine

catchers. Yes, it was obvious from looking

at all the other players, I was the ninth

catcher. I was basically just there to fill out

the roster and I realized if I ever wanted to

have a chance at a college career after my

freshman year, I would have to go through a lot of changes.

One of those changes was to improve my strength, size and fitness. Instead of going off and playing in the summer league after my freshman year, I got a job at a golf course. This was intentional because it forced me to get up every morning at five thirty in order to mow the greens. This meant I was done with work by 1:00 PM and provided plenty of time to spend on training. I would eat and immediately head to the weight room and lift for two hours.

After lifting, I'd go to a little rickety, church field with a bucket of balls. I'd throw ball after ball into the makeshift backstop (really just a fence) in lieu of long toss with a partner. Once I emptied the bucket, I'd pick up the balls and do it all over again. That's why when I hear a player say, "Hey I don't have a partner to throw with," to me it sounds like a poor excuse for not practicing. Hitting was a bit more of a challenge. The closest indoor hitting facility was about an hour drive from my home which ate up at least three hours a day, but I did it. That was my routine, day in and day out, during the summer between my freshman and my sophomore years of college. I was hoping the hard work paid off. When I arrived on campus at St. Andrews as a sophomore there were five catchers. During the early days of fall practice, I could tell my game had changed. Hits that barely made it to the outfield before, got to gaps for extra base hits. My teammates noticed the improvement in my arm strength and no one wanted to play catch with me. My daily routine was to play long toss and throw the ball as far as I could every day. Most players throw long toss a couple days a week, but very few push themselves to throw long toss for as long as they could every day. I transitioned through throwing partners every couple days. The joke became *if you want to throw long toss, throw with Chance.*

As the fall season wore on, we had our last testing period in which the entire team was timed in the 60-yard dash, which in my opinion is one of the most ridiculous and archaic tests of baseball skill utilized by both pro and college scouts to this day. Scouts have always stated that the 60 time is a measure of a player's athletic ability. A good time for a catcher in college would be 7.0-7.2. Anything under a 7.0 for a catcher would be considered above average. As noted earlier, I was slow, which meant, my foot speed and over all speed had become a priority that fall. I knew with my size and strength, I was never going to be a big power hitter so I figured if I could improve my speed, I could finagle my way into the lineup as a base running threat. All fall I focused on improving my speed with short sprints, long sprints, chasers (drills involving actually chasing another person), lunges and everything and anything I thought would help my foot speed and

agility. I needed to turn the coach's head.

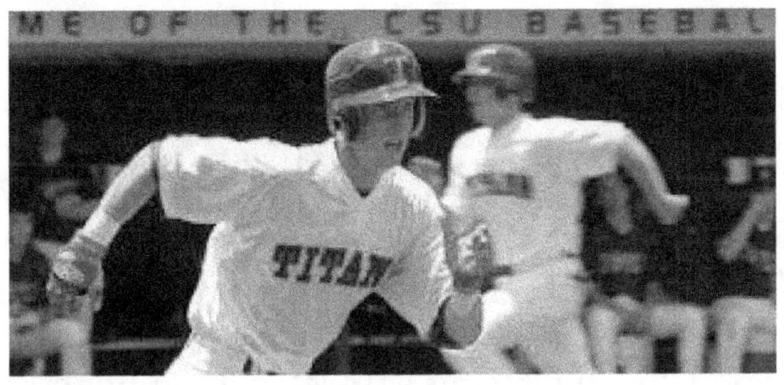

On the final day of testing I ran 60 yards in

6.8 seconds. The look on the coach's face

was priceless. Over the course of 18

months, from the spring of my senior year in

high school to the fall of my sophomore year

in college, I'd shaved a full second off my

best 60-yard time. I believe that was the first time the St. Andrews coaching staff ever really thought I had what it takes to be a serious college player. Still, as we broke for the winter, I wasn't exactly sure where I stood in the catching depth chart. When we returned for the spring semester it happened. The leading candidate to start for us that spring failed two classes and his parents refused to allow him to return to campus. Another catcher got home sick and decided to transfer over the break. Our catching staff went from five to three.

As we started the spring practices the guy who I had felt would be my greatest competition sprained his ankle playing basketball. I had my opening so I took it and never looked back. I ended up starting at catcher that spring. I hit .370, led the conference for all catchers in hitting and started again as a junior.

By any measure, I was enjoying an exceedingly successful college career at St. Andrews. The problem was on the inside. I struggled, I cried myself to sleep at nights, many nights, just because desperately I knew I was capable of pursuing NCAA baseball. I worked tirelessly and consistently day after day, week after week, to even have an opportunity to compete at the next level, much less to be the best. After my junior year I realized if I was going to have the chance to test myself at the next level, it was probably time for me to move on.

I ended up transferring to Lander University, an NCAA Division 2 school. Lander's new coach, Rust Stroupe, had recruited me out of High School to play for him at Brevard Junior College so I felt good about the move. I hadn't gone to Brevard Junior College out of High School because I had a case of *four-year-itis. Four-year-itis* is when a high school player, hell-bent on attending a four-year college, snubs junior college because he feels it is a lesser option. In retrospect I was that guy. I cared about what everybody else thought instead of what was best for me. What was best for me was going to junior college. I graduated at 17 years old. I was immature, under-sized and could have benefitted from the additional time to grow, get stronger and develop as a player at a junior college that Coach Stroupe was offering me. I truly believe that by

blowing off Coach Stroupe's offer to play at
Brevard, I made a huge mistake for no
reason other than I didn't know any better. I
like to think I could have ended up at a
bigger school if I didn't suffer from *four-year-itis.* I suppose I will never know, but I
share my experience with player after player
to help them not make the same mistake that
I did.

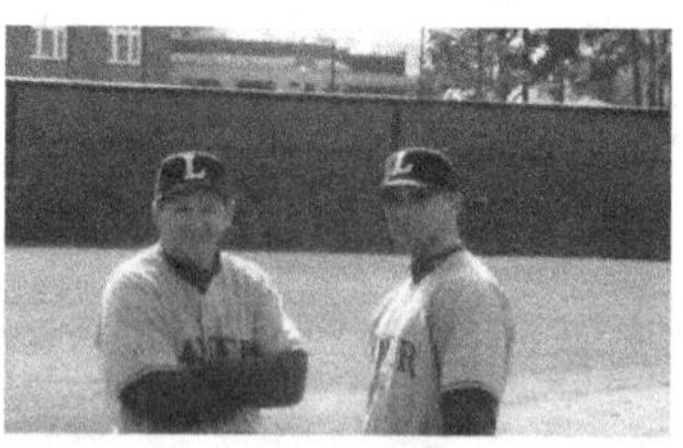

Coach Stroupe turned out to be a blessing in my life. He is a great

RUSTY STROUP AND ASST. COACH
CHRIS RODRIGUEZ - LANDER 1998

man, follower of Christ and steward of men.

I owe him a huge debt of gratitude for taking

a chance on me as a senior transfer in his

very first year at Lander University to start

his baseball program.

When I transferred from St. Andrews to

Lander I had come from an environment that

was toxic. Playing for Coach Swanson had

made me a man. It made me grow up and for

that I am grateful, but I left St. Andrews in

need of something. I wasn't certain what I

needed, but I knew it was something so I

reached out to Coach Stroupe, who had

recruited me to play at Brevard Junior College out of high school. It was this impulsive phone call to a coach I barely knew that changed my life. Coach Stroupe informed me that he had switched jobs and was now the head coach at Lander University. Coach Stroupe was not a loud man. He demanded excellence of his players, but he achieved it by setting a standard and allowing his upper classmen to drive the group. I was eager to take on this role of leadership under his guidance, particularly after having played under Coach Swanson, who was somewhat of a drill sergeant.

I was one of the only seniors that first year and was the very first senior to graduate from Lander University baseball program in 1998. Interestingly, we played University of South Carolina - Aiken at home in a game three-game conference series. I ended up going 7 for 13 that weekend and in the Sunday game Lander turned six double plays, setting the NCAA record for double plays in the same game, which I believe still stands today. The USC-Aiken coach got so mad after that sixth double play -which concluded with a bang-bang out at first – that he kicked the ball bucket and the balls scattered all over the field. It turns out that coach was the same guy who made it clear

to me four years earlier that I could never

play at that level. After the weekend series,

as we shook hands, I made sure to reminded

him that I was the same kid that he said

would never play at that level. He told me

no, but I had the last laugh on that one.

I was told no in junior high school, was told

no in high school, I was told no in college

and again I made liars out of every person

along the way.

After I graduated and played my last college game, I cried. I had forgone winter break for working out at gyms. I had never gone on one spring break trip. I had lived vicariously through MTV and all the people I had seen on TV enjoying their spring breaks and parties. I had spent countless hours hitting, lifting, running and eating to attain success at the college level, in the hopes that I would fill a void. A void of what I had I dreamed of from that very first time I hit that ball with my grandparents in their side yard.

I waited for the Major League Baseball amateur draft in June of 1998. I thought my baseball career was done. I didn't get drafted as expected, but I heard about an independent league called the Frontier League. Tryouts were in Chillicothe, Ohio on May 17 and 18. I drove the 6.5 hours from Lake Wylie, South Carolina to Chillicothe, Ohio for the Frontier League's league-wide tryout. I had no idea what the trip was going to hold, but I felt like a dead man walking as I laced up my cleats for the last time on that weekend in May. The tryout was a typical professional style tryout. More than 350 players ran the 60 yard- dash for time. Outfielders threw from right-field, infielders threw from second-base and catchers threw to second-base. I remember being the very first of around 25 catchers to throw. I wanted to set the bar high and imagined, as I prepared to throw, that I performed so well I became the standard to which every other catcher would be compared. Late on that first day of tryouts, my dad came by and wished me a happy birthday. I was so focused, I had completely forgotten it was my own birthday.

The second day consisted of a scrimmage.
With so many players present, you were
lucky to get one at-bat so it was difficult to
showcase your skills. This was very
frustrating. Late that afternoon the league
held its amateur draft. I attended knowing
my fate was probably all but set. The draft
began and as pick after pick was announced
I realized that no position players were
being taken, only pitchers. After the draft
concluded the Manager from the Johnstown
Johnnies walked down the middle isle of the
chairs that had been set up for the draft. I
had my head down as I made my way out. I
lifted my head and this tall skinny man,

lifted his hand to introduce himself to me. I had noticed him from the last two days of the tryouts, but couldn't place him as a coach, manager or player personnel from any of the teams that were in the league. He simply said, "Hi, I am Stephan Rapaglia, the manager of the Johnstown Johnnies." He went on to explain that the Johnnies, one of the teams in the Frontier league, had a tryout the next day at their stadium in Johnstown. He didn't promise me anything. He simple said he wanted to see more of me and invited me to the tryout.

My mother and my dad attended the second round of tryouts with me because, frankly, while unspoken, we all believed my playing days were coming to an end. We drove to Johnstown, Pennsylvania together, another five-hour road trip through countryside I'd never seen and proved to be not especially memorable.

I arrived at the field early. 11 or so players were there all by personal invitation. At the end of the day I approached the head coach, "Pags, so what do you think?" "Chance," he replied, "you did a good job. We start spring training tomorrow. I'd like to see you

there."

Every single day, for 11 straight days, I

woke up early thinking it might be the last

time I'd put on a pair of spikes as a player. I

was the first one to the field. I was the first

one to complete running and warm-ups. I

was the first to hit and first to help. I raked,

picked up trash, and every chance I got, I

hustled. One of the veteran independent

leaguers told me I needed to slow down

because it was a long season. Perplexed by

his advice I simply stated, "I am just trying
to make the ball club."

Each day, as players were released one by
one, I found myself hanging on. As spring
training came to an end, the coaching staff
was charged with making the last round of
cuts. Pags gathered the remaining 32 players
together for a pep talk before cutting down
to the final 24-man roster. I can't remember
what he said… only that the finality of my
fate was near. After he entered his office,
the three veterans, who knew they'd made
the team at that point, stood up and

announced they would be first. As the last of the veterans entered the coach's office, I stood up and said, "Guys, I lived every day for the last 11 days, as if it was my last day of playing baseball. I am going through that door next!" No one argued with me. As I exited the office door, all the players gathered around to hear me say, "I made it!" That moment was the was a culmination of a lifetime of blood, sweat and tears. I was showered with congratulations from men, some of whom were going home themselves. It felt as if I had been inducted into an exclusive fraternity, of which I am proud to be small part to this day.

I did not have a grand professional career. I didn't make millions of dollars, but looking back at my career, every person that said no along the way was put there at the exact moment I needed to add fuel to my fire. Don't take no as no. With the right attitude, a lot of effort and a little bit of MONA. No was my springboard into what came next every step of the way.

Inning #2 Why the Titans?

I began coaching college baseball in 2000, at the conclusion of my brief professional career. My first position was at North Greenville College in South Carolina as an assistant under Head Coach Tim Nihart. After one season at North Greenville, I was accepted into the Master of Business Administration program at the University of Tennessee, where I also landed a graduate assistantship under Coaches Rod Delmonico, Larry Simcox and Randy Mazey. Coaches Simcox and Mazey really took me under their wings during an

incredible season in Tennessee baseball

history.

Interestingly, I first met Randy Mazey (who

is currently the head coach at West Virginia

University) when I was a baseball camper at

Clemson University. He pitched at Clemson

for Coach Wilhelm and later became a

volunteer assistant coach. I kept in touch

with Coach Mazey from high school through

to the end of my pro career and it was this

relationship that got me the assistant

coaching opportunity at Tennessee. Coach

Mazey taught me the ropes of recruiting and coaching at the college level. He networked like no one I had ever met, making certain to say hello and exchange stories with as many coaches as possible on different staffs. He understood the baseball world was small and there was no telling who your next head coach might be or where your next opportunity was going to present itself.

That year UT finished third at the College World Series in Omaha and 13 members of the squad were taken in the 2001 Major League Draft. Most notably were first-round picks, Chris Burke and Wyatt Allen, who

both were great players and even better

people.

While completing my MBA at UT, I moved

to the assistant coaching position at Carson

Newman, a Division II college in Jefferson

City, Tennessee. It proved to be another

great coaching experience. The team was

conference champion's and outfielder Heath

Mason, was named All-American and

Division II Player of the Year. What an

incredible group of young men. Carson

Newman proved to be another great

coaching experience because I was able to

see excellence yet again at a championship

level for a second year. Even having had

only two jobs in two divisions, I joked that

no coach in the country had experienced

more success than me in my short career. In

spite of this success, however, I realized a

career in college baseball was not for me.

Young assistant coaches, many older than

me, whom I respected, shuffled from one

school to the next for poor salaries. Their

families struggled and personal lives

suffered as they pursued dreams of coaching

at the college level. Assistant coaches invested again and again in young men, poured themselves into fund raising and recruiting and often times were fired for things outside of their control. I came to the conclusion that I did not want that sort of life.

While I loved the game and found teaching and mentoring players to be very rewarding, I realized making a living as a college coach is no easy task. Head coaches in division I power conferences are paid well, but most coaches are starving… literally starving.

College coaches work long hours for very little pay and many work multiple jobs in order to support their families. I saw great people and coaches all struggling to make ends meet and decided that was not going to be my chosen career path.

My wife, Christine, who was my fiancé' at the time, took a leap of faith and moved with me to Marietta, Georgia where I took a job teaching high school. Six weeks into the school year I realized I was not cut out for teaching and promptly resigned my position and took a job in the mortgage industry. I had settled into my 9 to 5 job and was earning a comfortable living when I got a life changing phone call from a buddy of mine named Myles Shoda. At the time, Myles was the Braves' John Smoltz's agent and he was also deeply connected to the youth baseball scene in the Atlanta area. The purpose of his call was to coax me into coaching an East Cobb Baseball summer team.

East Cobb Baseball was founded in 1985 by Guerry Baldwin and was the preeminent travel baseball organization of the 1990's and 2000's. The program boasted its own facility with eight fields and sponsored approximately 85 teams ranging in age groups from 8U to 18U.

At first, I thought the idea of coaching youth baseball was an awful one. What could I possibly gain from coaching a bunch of sixteen-year-olds? I'd played professionally and coached at the college level after all and had decided coaching was not for me, but Myles was persuasive. After a good bit of arm twisting, I eventually agreed to give it a try.

At the end of that summer, Guerry Baldwin, owner of East Cobb Baseball, asked me if I was planning to coach again next year. I discussed the idea with Christine and being well acquainted with my baseball addiction, she encouraged me to pursue it. Initially my intention was for coaching youth baseball to serve as my stress outlet. Besides, it was just a summer youth team so how much time and energy could that take?

I began building my team in the fall of 2003. I had the tryout list with all of the names and numbers from the main tryout. The main tryout was held in early August. Times have changed, but back then ECB would have over 200 players come to the main tryout. The two days of the tryouts were long. I kept copious notes on all players. Who pitched? Who were the catchers? What were the players' actions? How did they run? Slow or fast? How big were they? Were they fat or strong, small or agile? After the tryout I would pour through these notes to try to put together a team.

When forming my team, one of the first

tasks was choosing a team name and

uniform colors. As is typical for youth

baseball programs, most of the East Cobb

Baseball teams were named after major

league ball clubs. Most notably were the

East Cobb Astros, East Cobb Yankees and

East Cobb Braves. Interestingly, my

professional baseball experiences were not

my most memorable. The greatest and most

positive experiences I'd had in all my years

in baseball took place during the time I spent

on the college diamond as both player and

coach. The camaraderie and fellowship I

shared with my college teammates, coaching

colleagues as well as the athletes I coached resulted in friendships that are proving to last a lifetime. It's no wonder one of my favorite college programs served as the inspiration for my team name.

When I was an assistant at the University of Tennessee, we opened the 2001 season with a road trip to Cal State Fullerton to play in a non-conference round robin tournament called the KIA Invitational. The other teams invited were Long Beach State and Wichita State, but I was as excited as a kid on Christmas day about playing Cal State

Fullerton because I'd been a life-long fan. When I was in high school especially, I really, really loved the way they played the game. The entire team always seemed to have a collective chip on its shoulder, and they were willing to take on the challenge of playing anyone. In the 1990's Cal State Fullerton was a perennial powerhouse. They made four College World Series appearances and won the national championship in 1995 under head coach, Augie Garrido. Augie Garrido was fiercely competitive and a passionate coach. He always seemed to be able to get the most out of his players. He set the tone for the program in the 90's that I believe lives on today. In the Spring of 2001, Tennessee baseball was ranked fifteenth in the country and Cal State Fullerton was ranked fifth. I was excited to see how we would fair. We were, after all, the big SEC opponent coming across country to play the small state directional school known only for baseball.

Well, not only did Cal State Fullerton have the audacity to believe that they could beat up on us, but they actually did beat up on us

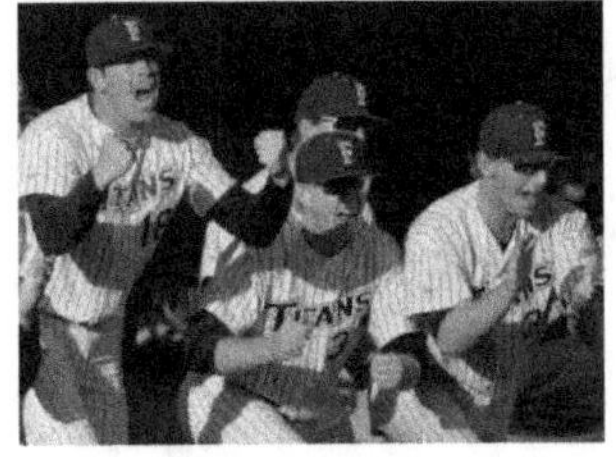

like there was no tomorrow. Later that

season, we ended up on the opposite sides of the bracket in the college world series in Omaha in 2001, but never got the chance to seek revenge. That 2001 team, and many to follow, was a phenomenal group of young men. They had great passion and respect for the game, and they played the right way. I just can't say enough great things about the Cal State Fullerton Titans and so, in 2003, when it came to selecting a name for my team, it was a no brainer and the East Cobb Titans was born.

Next on the docket was ordering uniforms. I decided I would stick with Cal State Fullerton's colors and so I ordered navy blue and bright orange. In fact, I have a very specific memory of telling Guerry Baldwin exactly what colors I wanted. I was wearing a navy-blue long-sleeved t-shirt and I vividly remember touching my sleeve and saying, "This blue." I also emphasized that the orange was not Texas-burnt orange, but bright orange, "just like Cal State Fullerton."

Imagine my surprise when months later

when I opened my box of uniforms to find

they were royal

blue and

orange…not

navy blue and

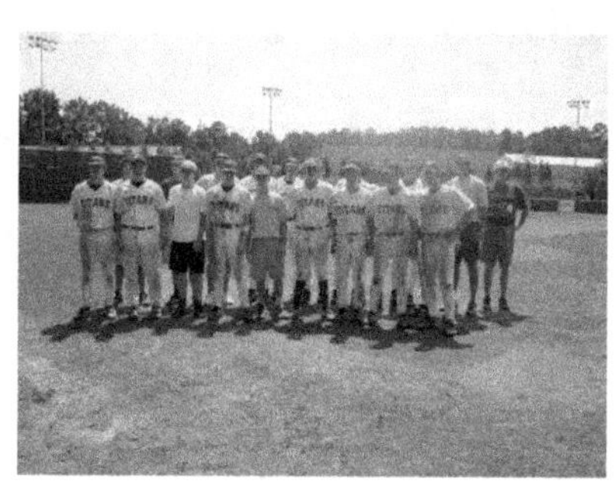

2005 TITANS

orange. It was bad

enough to have gotten the wrong color

uniforms, but there was probably no worse

color combination for a U of T alumnus

AND former member of the University of

Tennessee baseball staff! Why? Royal blue

and orange are the team colors for the

University of Florida Gators, Tennessee's

most contentious conference rivals. The

royal and orange of Florida makes many a

Tennessee fan physically ill. Needless to

say, I was not happy. Wearing Gator colors

was a bitter pill to swallow, but I did it and

the funny thing is, that was in 2003 and here

we are, 17 years later, still wearing royal

blue and orange. I guess everybody looks

good in Titan's royal blue and

orange…especially really good players!

Inning #3

Becoming an elite athlete is not an end goal, it is a process. This is not something of which I was fully aware when I started the Titans program in 2003. I had always thought of developing elite baseball players and coaching teams capable of winning National championships as reaching a destination. Rather than focusing on the process, I was focused on achieving the end goal. I imagined success to be like reaching a summit, as something like the end of a long road packed with hard work and determination; a place where everything was perfect. However, when I reached that "summit" it felt hollow and barren. I was perplexed. The success I had been aspiring to achieve for myself and players had arrived, but the feeling fell flat. Over time, I realized the value of the process was more gratifying and fulfilling than the end goal…the destination.

In 2003 when I started coaching youth baseball at East Cobb Baseball in Marietta, Georgia, the program was a travel baseball mecca. It was one of the only youth facilities in the country of its kind, with multiple

premier fields in one location. The program

was known for cultivating powerhouse

players and teams at every age level. Elite

teams from all over the United States, as

well as South and Central America, travelled

to ECB to play in high profile tournaments

in front of hordes of college recruiting

coordinators and pro scouts. It also was

common for talented players from all over

the United States to attend ECB try outs in

the fall with a plan to spend their summers

with local host families in order to play on

ECB teams. Since then, many other quality

youth baseball programs have popped up

around the country. Likewise, the number of premier facilities has increased.

Back in the early 2000's the prime recruiting season revolved around the Perfect Game World Wood Bat Association (WWBA) World Series tournaments hosted at ECB and typically lasted for three weeks. Tournaments consisted of the 16, 17 and 18-year-old age groups. Each age group lasted a full week and teams were guaranteed at least 7 games in pool play. The winner of each pool advanced to a single elimination bracket, with games played until the field was whittled down to the last two remaining

teams who then played each other in the

championship game. This type of event can

be described best as survival of the fittest,

with an undeniable advantage for teams with

the most quality arms and deepest pitching

rotations. So many games being played by

high level players in one location made ECB

fertile ground for recruiting. Literally

hundreds of college recruiters along with pro

scouts from all 30 major league

organizations flocked to ECB during that

three-week period every summer.

Nowadays, with showcase tournaments

including younger age groups, the summer

recruiting season starts around Memorial

Day weekend and extends through late

August.

Being part of East Cobb Baseball in the

early 2000's was a status symbol for players

and coaches alike. In 2003 alone, East Cobb

Baseball teams won a collective 11 National

Titles. Winning national championships was

expected. When I started the Titans in 2003,

we were just another team…another cog in

the wheel of East Cobb Baseball, but by

2006 we'd begun to earn our stripes as a

formidable team and as any coach will tell you, success starts with try outs.

As previously stated, tryouts for teams were held in early August each year at the main ECB facility in Marietta. Guerry Baldwin, the owner and director of East Cobb Baseball, coached the 16u ECB Astros and assigned himself the privilege of drafting his entire team before any other coached drafted a single player. Obviously, his teams were loaded with talent. Many of his players went on to be high level MLB draft picks and D1 college players in power conferences. It was not unusual during that time period for more than 200 players in each age group to show up for the two-day try-out. Each group could have as many as 12 teams. All of the coaches got a list of players on the morning of the draft. Due to the large number of players you had to be able to quickly note who you wanted and who you didn't. This was never more important than in the draft meetings at the end of day two of the tryouts.

The draft would start with Guerry calling out his list of names of the players he was selecting to take those players off the board. That usually started the scramble as that would lope off approximately 24 players off the list of players. These were always the best. The trick was trying to identify the next tier of players that were unpolished, had potential, had not grown yet, hustled more than everyone else, or had a chip on their shoulder. These were the group of players for whom the remaining coaches had to fight. In an ordinary draft, the teams would go one by one selecting players. In these meeting we would go down the player list and call names. Coaches would claim players as names were called. If more than one coach tapped a player, the debate began, which meant you had better be prepared with a solid argument for claiming that player. Dad coaches automatically got their sons and often exploited the angle that a player was "friends with his son" and "they wanted to play together" or "needed to carpool." Insert eye roll.

The draft meetings were vicious. In my early years at ECB, I approached draft meetings as a painful requirement. Inevitably, I would find myself ending up on the short end of the bargaining table. Some

dad-coach and I would draft the same kid,
but I'd always lose because said kid was his
son's best friend, etc. etc. etc. Then I'd go
through the same process with another
draftee, who I'd end up losing because said
kid was buddies with some dad-assistant-
coach's kid. And so on. And so on. And so
on. Kids and parents who are lifelong
friends are a package deal and blah blah
blah. There's no winning in daddy ball.
None. Draft night often drove me to using
the sort of expletive language one might
consider unbefitting of someone who works
with kids. You get the picture.

In the summer of 2004, we ended up with a

team that had been thrown together in this

typical haphazard manner. I worked

tirelessly with my guys. I tried forcing,

coercing, massaging, cajoling, teaching,

training, reprogramming, educating, beating

(metaphorically, of course) my stable of less

talented players into believing they could be

the contenders. We started the summer

season with a record of 4-7. We struggled at

basically everything. We did not execute

basics. We did not make routine plays on

defense and we were always behind on pitch

counts. We failed to put the ball in play consistently on offense. I vividly remember saying to the group, "We can't expect to be successful in the big things, when we aren't focused on the little things." Each player had to focus on their role and how each pitch could change that role. For example, if a pitcher gets ahead in the count -say the count is one ball, two strikes count (1-2) - all three outfielders should take two steps to the opposite field side. If it's a right-handed hitter the outfield takes two steps toward the right field line. The reason for this is to re-position the outfield in such a way as to defend a more tentative hitter. Meanwhile, the corner infielder should take two to three

steps back to cover more ground. The

reason for this is with the hitter now having

two strikes the bunt is no longer an option.

The middle infielder can player deeper as

well now that the corner infielders are

playing deeper. This allows them to the

play the pitch being called instead of just

their portion of the field. So, if the catcher

calls a curveball on a 1-2 pitch, the shortstop

and middle infielder can move two to three

steps toward the first baseline for this right-

handed hitter to compensate for the tentative

hitter due to the count and the location of the

pitch as it will more than likely be thrown

down and away. These are the little things that every player has to focus on. When you begin to address these little things, the big things take care of themselves. The fly balls always seem to be within reach, the ground balls always seem to be routine.

As mid-summer unfolded, the guys got it. They started to play hard, they started to execute and they started to beat far more talented teams because they bought into the idea of doing all of the little things we had been working so hard on. One of the final tournaments of the season was the Perfect game World Wood Bat Associations 17u World Series. Going into the event there was a huge write up about a team from northern California called NorCal. They were loaded with 19 division 1 commits. They were ranked number 1 in the country by Perfect Game and were the odds-on favorite to win the entire tournament. After reading the article posted on Perfect game's site, I went about checking to see what our schedule for the week would be. Wouldn't you know it, we were slated to play NorCal in pool play. Which was great and awful all at the same time. In Perfect Game tournaments, teams have to win their pool to advance to championship play, but I noticed

that our pool seemed to have more teams in

it than the other pools. I shrugged it off

without much thought.

We started the week by winning our first

four games of the seven that were scheduled

for the week. We played some incredible

competition from all over the United States,

including teams from Texas, Pennsylvania

and Florida. Game five was our deciding

game with NorCal. I knew it was a different

atmosphere before the game even started.

When I got there the first three people at the

game were Major League Baseball scouts.

That's usually a good sign that someone

playing in the game is really good.

Knowing what we had on our roster, a great

group of college players for sure, I knew

that they hadn't come to watch us.

We played great and ended up losing 4-3 in

a nail-biter. That's right, I said it was a

great game and we lost. That may sound

odd, but I never talk about winning the

game. We talk about winning the pitch, the

inning, or an at bat. Never the game,

because you can't win games without

winning more pitches, innings and at bats

than the other team. NorCal had one more

run than we had when the game was over.

After the game I talked to my team and

encouraged them on their efforts and told

them how proud I was of them. On my way

out of the ball park, one of the coaches from

NorCal said, "Hey coach, great team you

have there." I said, 'Thanks not bad for a

16u group." His eyes seem to bulge out of

his head, "Sixteen!" he exclaimed. I

chuckled and explained we were playing up

an age class, but our week was basically

over after being handed a one run loss. He

said "Coach you may want to go back and

look at the rules for this tournament. Our

pool has more teams in it than the others, so

two teams from our pool advance to the

championship bracket." Sure enough, he

was right! I looked at our two remaining

pool games. The last pool game was against

the defending national champions, the

country's number-seven-ranked Orlando

Scorpions. We started that game on shaky

ground, getting down two runs early, but

battled back to make it a 6-5 game. With

two outs and two runners on base in the

seventh inning, Roman Grimaldi came to the

plate and hit a chopper between the first and

second baseman. Both runs score and we

won the game by a score of 7-6. It was an incredible feeling that this group of players had come so far in such a short period of time. After we shook hands, a Perfect Game representative found me in the crowd and asked me to come to a coaches meeting. Completely oblivious, I soon realized the coaches' meeting was for all the teams who had won their pool, or in our case came in second. I wasn't sure if I should just be happy my team had come this far, or if we had more to accomplish. As the Perfect Game staff fanned the room looking for coaches and announcing match ups, I hear *Titans play Perfect Game National.* I thought I heard the announcement wrong, as

I look at the guy next to me and said, "Did

he says Perfect game National?" He nodded

at me with a look of pity. I am sure he was

thinking, "Poor schmuck!"

Back in the early 2000's, Perfect Game

assembled their own national teams. This

particular team was ranked third in the

country. They didn't have two guys from

the same state, much less the same town. As

I collected myself after finding out whom

we were playing, I noticed that the coach of

the PG National team happened to be

standing to my right. I asked him, "You guys are really good apparently, what is your record?" He says, "55 and 1." In that moment, I probably would have been better served to just stay quiet, but of course, I didn't. As I turned to walk down the stairs to go out to the game, I said, "I hope you don't mind being 55-2."

We started the game against the Perfect National team about a half an hour after the coaches meeting ended. We hadn't gotten a single out in the first inning and we were already down 3-0. The weight of that comment was palpable as I walked out to the mound to make an early inning pitching change. We got out of the inning and things settled down. By the fifth inning we were still trailing 3-1, which was pretty respectable given our shaky start. I could see the PG National team starting to get a bit uncomfortable as they were used to run ruling most of the teams they played and never played in many close games. We hit six consecutive doubles in the fifth inning and our rallying cry became *take the fight to them!* When the dust settled… we won.

After the game a local newspaper reporter interviewed me about the game. He asked me specifically about the huge outburst we had in the fifth inning. I can't remember exactly what I said, but it was something along the lines of, "We prepare for those moments all the time." I laugh at that statement. I am not sure I have ever had a team hit six consecutive doubles since. Apparently, I am not doing a very good job of preparing players in comparison to my much younger self.

In the final game of the day, this rag tag group of guys who started the season 4-7 were in the Elite 8 of the Perfect Game

World Wood Bat Association 17u World

Series …as a 16u team. Who would be our

final match-up of the day? NorCal! I am

not sure who was more shocked me or my

players at having to play NorCal, ranked

number one nationally, for a second time in

three days. I was certain that if they had

taken us lightly in the previous game, they

wouldn't this time. We started the game

with a lefty by the name of Kyle Green.

Kyle weighed approximately 135 pounds.

He had knobby knees and elbows. He could

pitch, but it was not fast. The lead-off hitter

came to the plate and Kyle's first pitch,

barely breaking the speed limit on most

interstates, registered 69 miles per hour on the radar gun. The hitter swung fast and furious as the ball softly drifted past the hitter for strike one. It was comical to me and most of the people watching the game, but not to NorCal. I heard comments that we needed to throw the ball harder, so that they could hit it fair. I had anticipated this. I rallied the team and screamed, "Take the fight to them boys!" In retrospect I am sure there was many onlookers, thinking that I was some sort of a mad man, and it was clear that it was only a matter of time before the mighty NorCal would bring an onslaught of runs. But they didn't! Fast forward to the top of the seventh inning. NorCal is ahead with a 3-2 lead. We had runners on second and third base with two outs. NorCal brought in their closer. This was not just any closer. He was 6'5" and had topped out at 95 mph earlier in the week. He was projected to be a top three round pick in the Major League draft out of high school the following year. As he walked from the bull pen I watched pro and college scouts along with spectators from all over the park settle into the bleachers at our field to watch the spectacle David versus Goliath. A game where a no named team was taking the number one ranked team in the country to the final inning…and they had a chance. As the closer from NorCal warmed up, the hitter due up to the plate was our second baseman named Ryan Tinkoff. He was a switch hitter, but saying he was a switch would indicate he could hit from both sides of the plate. He could not. The closer was right-handed so Tink, as he was known to me and his teammates, said, "Coach, he's right-handed I am going to hit lefty." I said, "Tink, you've got no shot lefty. Go up and hit righty." I'll never forget what he says next, "I'll prove you wrong" with a huge smile. My response was, "You better start your swing now!"

Tink battled his way to a 1-2 count. He

somehow made solid contact and the ball

flared over second base and both runs

scored, shifting the score to 4-3 in our favor.

The team, parents and people I had never

seen before we cheering and celebrating this

bag of misfits' success. The closer recorded

the next out on three straight strikes. In the

bottom of the seventh, the lead-off for

NorCal hit a soft flyball down the right field

line. I saw where the ball landed and I

swear it was foul. The hitter thought it was

foul as well and ended up only getting to

first base. I called time and sprinted to the

right field line where the poor soul who was

the umpire stood. I proceeded to unleash a

tirade (unjustly I am certain), but I was not

going to allow anyone to take this moment

from my guys much less a missed call.

After a few minutes of my blowing hot air in

the field umpires’

direction, he tossed me. He threw me out of

the game! Most would have thought I had

truly lost it in that moment. No one would

have expected to happen what happened

next. I smiled and said, “Thanks!” I ran

back to mound and waved all my players on

the field to come to the mound. I explained

to them that I'd gotten tossed because I had

their backs and now I needed for them to get

three outs. Not for me, but for themselves.

It redirected

their focus to

what mattered

most. Get

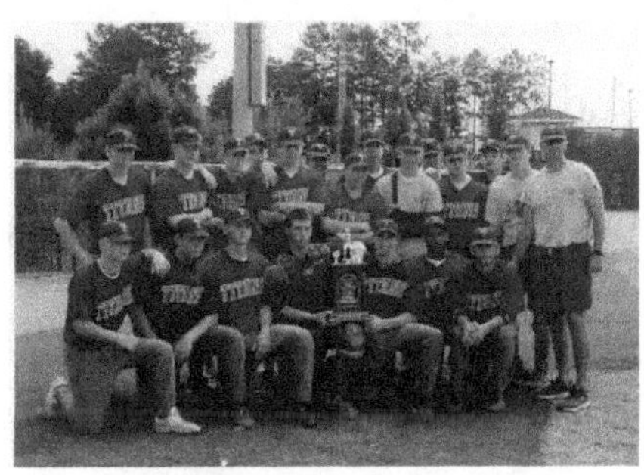

three outs. Not the emotion. They got three

outs! We won 4-3, finishing a day where

my band of misfits beat the numbers seven,

three and number one ranked teams in the

country in one day. In the semi-final, the

next morning, we got handled easily by the

eventual tournament champions, Kyle

Chapman from Texas.

I could not have been prouder of those

young men. They were my original Titans

and they played like Titans! If you look

very closely at our logo in our facility today

in the area of the 1TAT you can see this

group of young men.

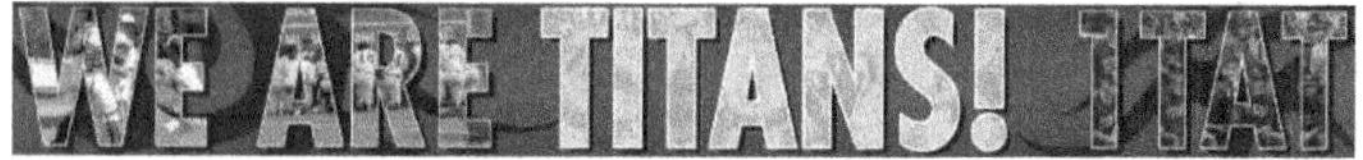

In 2005 we had considerable success, but I

watched many of the kids I wanted to take

from the previous year flounder on other

teams and their parents openly comment that

they wished they'd had an opportunity to

play for the Titans again. As the 2005

season drew to an end, I told Guerry

Baldwin I was done coaching. He asked

why and I explained that although I loved

coaching,
loved the
game and
oddly enough

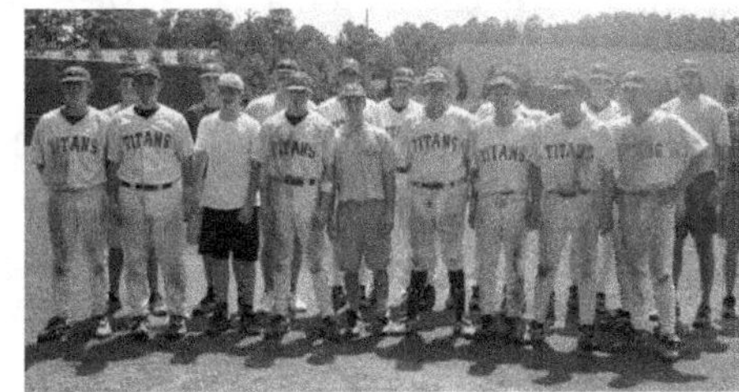

2005 TITANS

I even enjoyed spending my summers on the

field with a bunch of annoying adolescents, I

refused to lose players to a bunch of dad

coaches who resorted to playing the "but

he's my son's best friend" trump card. I

talked. Guerry listened. He promised to take

122

care of me in the upcoming draft for the 2006 season and ultimately, he convinced me to say on at East Cobb.

When August try-outs rolled around, I approached the process with cautious optimism, hoping that Guerry would keep his end of the bargain. Try-outs came and went in 2006 and Guerry kept his promise. I was allowed to have the second pick of the entire draft. Guerry would select his players, then the Titans got to pick their group of players. It was the first time I truly had a chance to pick my own team without interference. Overall, players on my 2006

team were the most talented I'd had. In

essence, the Titans became the number two

team at ECB in 2006. It felt good to receive

that nod from Guerry Baldwin. He had

confidence in me and although we were the

number two team, I held myself and my

players to the same standard that Guerry set

for the Astros. I expected my team to win

year in and year out. While being the

number two team out of ECB was certainly

something of which to be proud, we also

played with a bit of a chip on our

shoulders. Looking back, the level of talent on Geurry Baldwin's Astros was staggering. I should never have expected the Titans to play at their level and I thank God for my naivety back then because somehow by His grace, we did!

That year, I had a group of incredibly talented young men, I challenged them in ways many of them had never before been challenged. I remember one stretch of the season in particular that was a grueling test of not only physical and mental ability, but of character. We played 12 games in six days. I'd entered the team in a league in Nashville, Tennessee hosted by a friend and all-around great human being, Mikey Hiter. League rules mandated we complete our regular season league games by a certain date. Unfortunately, we had a lot working against us as we tried to get all our games played. I was still working as a mortgage broker at the time and had difficulty getting enough personal time off to make weekend trips to Tennessee and Alabama. When I could get the needed time off, our opponents had schedule conflicts. Inclement weather played havoc with our local and home game schedules and we ultimately found ourselves with the play-by date looming and a lot of catching up to do. Forfeiting was not an option so I did what any coach would do. I set the schedule - 12 games in six days including travel to and from two states – and announced it to the players and parents. Not a single person batted an eye-lash or uttered a word, but in retrospect, I'm certain they thought I'd lost my mind.

We started those grueling six days in Marietta by playing doubleheaders on Tuesday, Wednesday, and Thursday. We packed up after Thursday's games and travelled to Tullahoma, Tennessee where

played a Friday night doubleheader. On

Saturday we moved onto Nashville for our

fifth doubleheader. On Sunday we travelled

to Auburn, Alabama for our final

doubleheader of that painful stretch. We

played 12 games in six days and went 11-1.

That group of young men was incredible. I

was extremely proud of them.

I believe one of the main reasons this team

was able to achieve all they did was

because they believed in me and each other.

They looked around the dugout and saw

their teammates giving it their all daily.
They saw that as the head coach I didn't
allow myself to take days off mentally. I
didn't allow the top player or last player on
the roster to play by different standards.
They became a brotherhood through their
dedication, attitude and effort. We finished
the season winning our last game with a
final record of 61 and 19.

We wrapped up that summer season with
two high profile tournaments, the CABA
World Series and Super 7, both held at East
Cobb. We won the CABA World Series by

beating the Puerto Rican National Team in the semi-finals and an excellent team from Ohio in the finals. The final week of the season was reserved for the Super Seven World Series. Teams invited to the Super Seven World Series were considered to be the top seven 16u travel teams in the country. We were honored to be included in an event that crowned the best of the best. We played teams from all over the country, from California to Florida and found ourselves in the championship game, facing none other than Guerry Baldwin's ECB Astros. The Titans were exhausted from playing 80 games over the course of 90 days. This last game of the season certainly seemed to be our final test. Both teams played the game with passion and determination. In the end we won, beating my mentor Guerry Baldwin's team by a score of 5-2. The elation we felt is indescribable. We finished that season with two National Titles and a final record of 61 and 19.

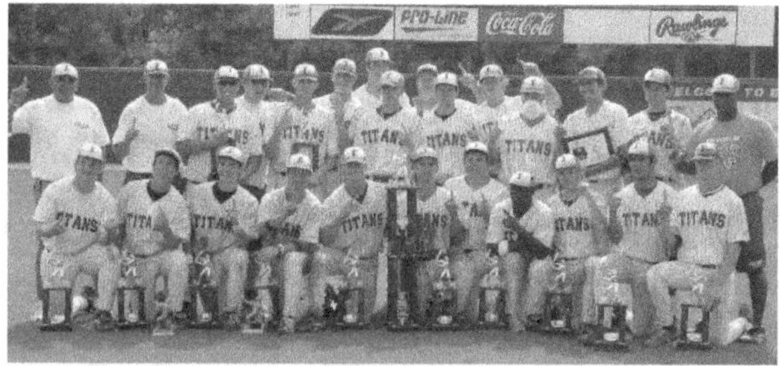

TITANS 2006

Out of 18 players on that Titans roster, 11

players went on to play college baseball.

Andy Marinelli played at Georgia State.

Taylor Black played at ABAC, which is a

Division III school. Marcus Grimaldi played

at Liberty. Evan Martin played at Georgia

Tech. Chris Base played at Armstrong

Atlantic State, which was a Division II

school at the time. Matt Skole played at

Georgia Tech and is now playing

professional baseball with the Chicago

White Sox organization. Scott Haddock

played at Piedmont, a Division III school in

Georgia. Jared Northcutt played at Barry

University. Brad Moss played at Sanford

University, went on to play professionally in the San Francisco Giants organization and is now coaching at the University of Montevallo. Jonathan Harris played at Gardner Webb University, had a stint in the professional ranks and is now coaching at Reinhardt University. Elliot Byers played at Stanford. They were simply an extraordinary group of young men and I am so proud of every single one of them. I am honored by the thought that I might have played some small part in shaping them into the fine men they have become today.

I still consider that summer season to be the pinnacle of success in my travel baseball coaching career, but once it ended, I was a bit lost. For weeks, I could not seem to find my bearings. When it all began in my mind, the goal was to win a national championship. I had only thought about winning that national championship. I had placed my own self-worth on winning that trophy. In hindsight, I measured success by attaining a measly trophy. I remember being very preoccupied about what people thought of me and if I led a team to win a national championship what that would mean.

Looking back, I realize that it was a great

accomplishment that will always be a fond

memory. However, what I did find through

the weeks after winning that national title

was achieving a goal is not what fulfils me.

It's the process of striving for perfection

each day.

I reflected on what my thoughts about those

same players would have been if we had lost

those games? Would their efforts have been

any less? If we had lost the National

Championship games in that particular

season, would the season be a failure? This

is where I started really questioning myself

for putting so much emphasis on winning and losing. Just because we won those games doesn't mean that the season was a success. In the same way, if we would have finished, 59 and 21, would that entire season be a failure because we lost the two national championship games? This really made me start to question the idea of what a champion really is. What does it really mean? The team attained what I had driven them to do all summer and now what?

I had no clue what to shoot for next. I had a bit of an identity crisis after the season for almost eight weeks. I would find myself

turning the radio off driving down the road

saying to myself out loud, "You have won a

National Championship, now what?" At

times I thought that I just needed to quit

coaching all together. I had achieved what I

had set out to do. Then another part of me

would speak out, "Are you that shallow?

You only coached for some dumb trophy?"

I was filled with mixed emotions of relief,

confusion and anxiety. Relief for being able

to achieve what many thought couldn't be

done. Winning a National Championship

and beating Guerry's team in so doing.

Confused because suddenly I didn't know

what to do next. And anxious because I had

never questioned my future in baseball.

Baseball marked the times of my life.

I was really trying to wrap my mind around

what had happened. Because I had always

been the player that wasn't quite good

enough, wasn't strong enough and always

had to work harder and focus more, as a

coach, experiencing that level of success for

the first time with one of my teams was

disorienting. I realized that winning games

and becoming an elite athlete is a by-product

of a certain mindset. I call it a winning

attitude. I realized that it wasn't the goal of winning a National Championship that had driven me. It was the idea of that goal. It was the pursuit of perfection and pursuit of excellent execution. It was the process.

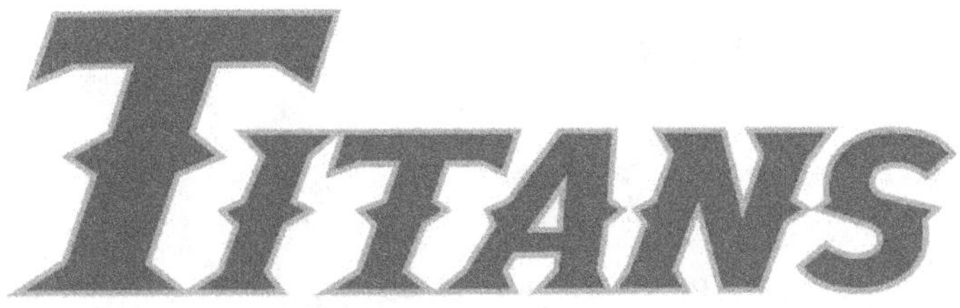

College recruiting?

Come and see what we offer for our players and see why we have had more than 700 players go on to play college or professional baseball.

TitansNation.net/College-Program

Inning #4 The Seed

By spring of 2008, the Titans had grown from one team to four teams. Per usual, we drafted our 16U roster and added a 9U, 10U, 11U team. The whole Titans thing was still a hobby for me, but my reputation as a coach and developer of quality players was growing so folks with younger kids began looking to the Titans for travel ball opportunities. It didn't surprise me that parents of these younger players were excited about making a Titans team, but what I didn't expect was their enthusiasm for spirit wear. Remember, my prior Titans had only ever been 16U. The parents I'd encountered up to that point had never expressed any desire for spirit wear, but parents of our newly minted 9U, 10U and 11U team members not only wanted spirit wear, they expected it in an array of sizes and styles suitable for outfitting Junior's entire cheering section - mom, dad, brother, sister, grandma and grandpa – in coordinating t-shirts, shorts, caps and visors.

In 2008, I was a full-time mortgage banker. Many of my professional colleagues took up golf or tennis to relax. Others spent their

summers boating and fishing, but my hobby

was coaching baseball. My hobby was the

Titans. I wore a suit and tie

every day and looked forward to unwinding

on the baseball field, but when these parents

began making requests for spirit wear, my

hobby was growing less relaxing by the

minute. I didn't have any gear because there

had never been a demand for it, so I reached

out to a guy by the name of Steve Vogel, a

sales rep with a sports apparel company call

Aladame, to inquire about ordering some

customized spirit wear. He collected some

information and put together a proposal.

We met at a little table in the breakfast area

of the Spring Hill Suites by Marriott in

Kennesaw, Georgia.

We discussed t-shirts,

hats and other spirit

items. Steve went over

quantities, sizes, prices

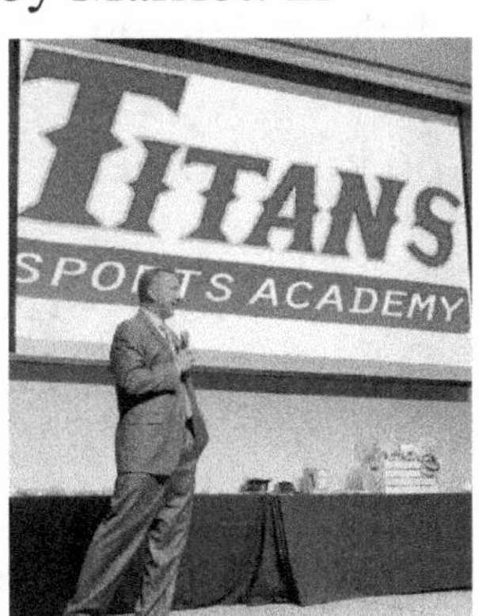

BANQUET 2019

and finalized delivery and payment details.

As the meeting was drawing to a close,

Steve started putting all his paperwork back

into this manila envelope so I began to do

the same. As I packed up my notes and pens, Steve looked over at me and said, 'Chance, what are you doing?" I'll never forget that moment. There was this long pause and then my response, "Steve, what do you mean what am I doing? I'm ordering stuff, um, you know, ordering spirit wear and putting my stuff away." He said "No, Chance. What are you doing with this Titan thing?" I'll never forget he just called it "this Titan thing." I paused. I vividly recall staring out the window by the table where we had been sitting and asking him again what he meant. He explained that there wasn't really anyone else who was growing his own brand within the East Cobb organization and wondered

what I was doing. I remember he just looked

at me incredulously as if to say what are you

trying to do? I really don't even remember

what I said, I don't know. But that

conversation and the surrounding details

stuck in my head.

When I left that meeting, I felt like I'd been

bitten by a bug. I kept shaking my head and

thinking to myself what, what, what am I

doing? That conversation consumed my

every thought. Over the ensuing nights and

weeks, I found myself waking up thinking

about what defined the Titans and what it all

meant. I started asking myself what it would

look like if I truly created my own

organization. I even started having dreams

about a building with blue walls. I had no

idea what blue walls meant. Why would

they need to be blue, anyway? Everything

was royal blue, the walls were royal blue

from top to bottom, from the floor all the

way to the ceiling. There were signs as well,

but I couldn't really tell what the signs said.

I just had these recurring dreams about

Titans teams at different age groups with

multiple coaches and an evolving

organizational structure. All these ideas

started formulating in my head and I didn't really know where to place them because I had only ever thought of coaching youth baseball as a hobby. The Titans were my hobby. That's what I thought…

To this day, Steve Vogel has a very special place in my heart for a meeting he probably does not even remember. He has a special place in Titans' history because on that particular day, in April 2008, he planted the seed for an idea that would eventually grow into the reality that is Titans Sports Academy. As odd as it may sound, that meeting changed my life. In a single moment "this Titans thing" went from being my hobby to my vision and my passion and my mission so to you, Steve Vogel, I say thank you. Thank you, sir.

NOTE: Shortly after that day I was in a local Jimmy Johns sub shop and happened to read a sign that was hanging on the wall, "Don't give up on something you really want." It was one of the many affirmations I received in those days that kept me focused on my goal.

Inning #5 1TAT

The 2008 16U Titans were a formidable
team. All 11 of our starting pitchers threw
over 85 miles per hour. Andrew Smith, who
later pitched at University of North
Carolina, Ryan Newell who pitched in the
Marlins Organization, and Johnny Magliozzi
who pitched at the University of Florida and
in the Mets Organization anchored a
pitching staff which led the team to the
Fletcher World Series National
Championship. The championship game was

held at Tropicana Field, home of MLB

American League Tampa Bay Rays.

Johnny Magliozzi came

to East Cobb from East

Milton, Massachusetts

where he attended the

Dexter School in Boston

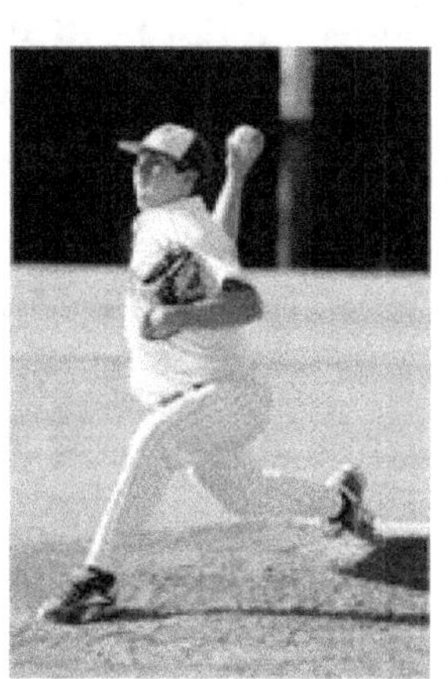

JOHNNY MAGLIOZZI 2008

and played baseball for

Dan Danato. He was ranked number two in

Massachusetts and 74th in the nation in the

2011 Final Class Rankings by Perfect Game

and was drafted straight out of high school

by the Tampa Bay Rays in the 35th round of

the 2011 Major League Baseball Draft.

Johnny decided to forgo signing a

professional contract in favor of attending

the University of Florida, in order to

continue his education and to be a part of a

perennial power house baseball program.

In December of his freshman year in

college, Johnny decided to visit a friend out

of town over a long weekend. In typical

Magliozzi fashion, he had concocted a plan

where he would be able to get out of town

and fly back in time for his mandatory

Monday morning lifting session at 6AM with the strength staff.

Unfortunately, his plans took an unexpected turn as the first leg of Johnny's flight back to Gainesville was delayed due to snow. He ended up missing his connecting flight in Atlanta and realizing he was in jeopardy of missing his lifting session, panic set in. Magliozzi had recently downloaded a new app to his phone called Facebook. Remembering most of his former teammates from the Titans lived and attended college in the Atlanta area, the resourceful young man jumped on the app and started messaging his

former Titans teammates for help.

Greg Bowder, who played with Magliozzi in

2008 and was in school at Georgia State

University in midtown answered the

message. He got up, drove 45 minutes from

the GSU campus to Harstfield-Jackson

Airport, retrieved his former teammate in

the middle of the night and delivered him to

a Greyhound Station where he hopped a bus

back to Gainesville. Evidently, Magliozzi

made it back to Florida in time for his 6am

weight lifting workout, but rumor has it the

weary traveler may not have woken up in
time to actually go.

The story of Greg Bowder's rescuing of
Johnny Magliozzi spread quickly among
members of the 2008 team and inspired the
tag line "Once a Titan Always a Titan." It

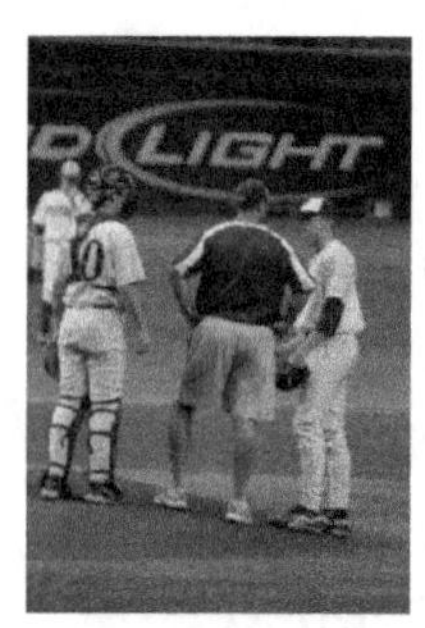

was shortened to 1TAT on
Facebook and eventually to
#1TAT on Twitter. #1TAT is
an unintended benefit of being

MOUND VISIT
2008 WS AT
TROPICANA PARK

a Titan. Teammates are
connected by a single summer filled with
perseverance, sweat, determination, success

and failure, the privilege of wearing a blue hat and orange jersey. The privilege of wearing the iconic blue cap includes an important mandate: it must ALWAYS be worn forward facing out of respect for the game and to honor all Titans… past…present…and future.

Inning #6 The ~~East Cobb~~ Titans

From 2003 to 2009, my tenure as coach of the East Cobb Titans, the East Cobb Baseball program was the mecca of the youth travel baseball world and I confess, albeit a part-time gig, it was also the focal point of my life. Sure, I was a full-time mortgage banker, but coaching kids filled a void for this self-proclaimed baseball junky. As an account executive for a mortgage lender, my job was to call on small to mid-size mortgage brokers and loan officers who represented clients seeking to secure loans to refinance or purchase homes. I also underwrote loans agreements and structured their funding from the portfolio of mortgage products my company offered. During this time there was a huge financial boom in the housing industry, which unfortunately led to the housing bust in 2008.

On December 30, 2008, the Case–Shiller home price index reported the most significant price drop in its history. The ensuing credit crisis resulted from the bursting of the housing bubble due to bad mortgage lending practices employed in the years leading up to 2009. Credit and funding for mortgage loans tightened up and my ability to close loans, and earn commissions, came to screeching halt.

During the summer of 2009, I coached the 16u Titans and managed three additional Titans teams in different age groups at East Cobb Baseball, all while still struggling to earn a living in the mortgage industry. Christine, my wife, went back to work to help make ends meet and I began to contemplate a career change.

I was desperate to make something work. I started a web design company with a friend of mine from Tampa, Florida. We had a team in India build the sites to control cost. Meanwhile I was also cross selling all my leads I was calling on merchant services. Of course, baseball was in the mix of potential options and it was at this point that I approached Guerry Baldwin, President of East Cobb Baseball, to discuss the possibility of my managing the ECB Academy. from his son and another part-time ECB staffer, who had been running it since its inception.

A typical day was to wake up at 6 AM and help Christine get the kids ready for day care. Next I was off to work to make my calls for my mortgage account executive position. By midday I was making other sales calls on the websites business I was simultaneously trying to start and sell merchant services. At 3:00 PM I would make my way to East Cobb to start this newfangled idea of an Academy. By 9PM I was finally home, but then would jump on video conference calls with our group in India to answer questions on the sites we had in progress. I would finish those calls

up at 3:00 AM and do it all over again the

next day. I hoped that ECB Academy would

catch on and become my priority. I think at

that point I was just trying to find a way to

pay the bills.

ECB Academy was created to be the

instructional arm of the East Cobb Baseball

program. Offering private lessons and off-

season camps was a great way to improve

players' skills and provided an opportunity

to increase revenue, but unfortunately the

ECB Academy never really got off the

ground. Guerry's son was a silent owner and his partner in the endeavor, an ECB staffer, was over extended and simply could not devote the time or energy required to operate the Academy and see it to its full potential.

Guerry accepted my proposal and in the fall of 2009, I purchased the "franchise" of ECB Academy. I still shake my head at the amount I paid for the right to give lessons and run camps at ECB. In retrospect, it was a hefty price to pay, but I   learned invaluable lessons in how run a thinly margined business. By middle May, 2010, I

had driven the academy business to the

threshold that made me ready to transition

out of the mortgage and banking industry,

website design and merchant services

business and into full-time career as a

baseball instructor and coach. With the

financial and emotional support of my wife,

along with her confidence and guidance, I

resigned from my mortgage job and leaped

head-first into East Cobb Baseball!

By summer of 2010, I was a fixture at the

complex. I was there every day running a

camp of some kind, managing my own private lesson calendar as well as the calendars of every ECB instructor giving private lessons at Academy, and running the Titans program with its ever-increasing band of teams. I had a solid working

relationship with Guerry Baldwin and the entire management staff at ECB. By fall 2011, work was complete on the expansion of the ECB indoor training facility. The building, nestled behind one of the premier fields inside the park, was to be shared by patrons of ECB Academy for camps and lessons and by East Cobb Baseball teams for batting and bullpen practices. This newly

expanded indoor facility would give the

ECB Academy a place to call home and the

increased square footage allowed for

expansion of the private lesson side of the

business. Initially I couldn't believe the

massive break I'd caught for myself and the

ECB Academy, but in retrospect it marked

the point at which I knew I eventually would

need to leave ECB.

With the new building came a new contract.

I came to the table ready to negotiate an

agreement to include, among other items,

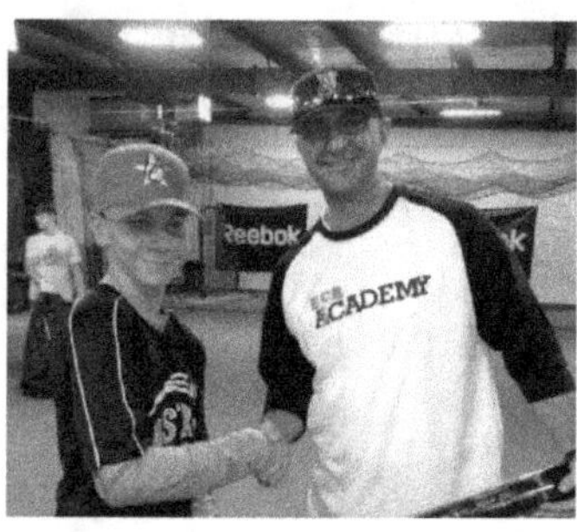

our use of the new

facility. In the

negotiations,

however, Guerry

included all of the

old parameters to which we'd previously

agreed, but he refused to include the new

ones I was requesting. There was also a 120

day out clause, where either party could, at

any point, opt out of the contract with no

cause. In addition, the new contract did not

grant me exclusivity for lessons and camps

at East Cobb Baseball. I understand

Guerry's reluctance to include my terms, but

it was a disappointment that prompted a

serious examination of my situation. The

seeds of discontent eventually led me to

decide to leave East Cobb Baseball, but it

would be two years before that decision

came to fruition.

To the outsiders I was the face of the ECB

Academy, and cheerleader for the program

and took pride in carrying the ECB flag onto

the field of play each summer. Negotiating

the new contract, however, made me realize

that I was never going to be accepted as a

real part of the inner sanctum of East Cobb

Baseball. Sure, I could function under their

banner so long as I kept writing monthly

checks to rent the name.

I had been loyal to the ECB brand, but I

realized that loyalty was not reciprocal and

it gave me reasons for concern. Sure, ECB

was the established leader in youth baseball

programs and the academy enjoyed a steady

flow of clientele, but it was now in writing

that at any point in time I could have

everything I'd work toward stripped away

from me in 120 days. A leadership change, a

disagreement, a difference of opinion or,

under the terms of the new contract even

nothing at all, is all it would take for me to

be left out in the cold. With a wife and

family to provide for, this was simply a risk

I was unwilling to take. I weighed my

options for nearly two years before making a

move, but in the summer of 2013, I finally

decided to sever ties with East Cobb

Baseball, Inc.

As I prepared to make a move, I noted
Guerry Baldwin and I hadn't had a
conversation in months. The tension
between us was at an all-time high. I had
much to do to ensure the nine Titans teams
formed under the East Cobb name would be
able to make the jump with me if the
program was going to survive. I knew the
players and their families would not leave
ECB without an indoor facility to call home.
Coincidentally, John Flading, owner of
Swing Away Sports products was looking
for someone to take over the lease on a
20,000 square foot indoor facility he had
secured, but no longer wanted or needed.

John and I met on several occasions to discuss the details of my taking over his lease. On one of those occasions, shortly before signing the contract, the stress of finalizing the decision to go out on my own had hit an all-time high. I recall sitting on a roll of turf at the facility while John and I were having a conversation about what was going to happen next. I got quiet and John asked, "What are you so worried about?" My response was not that I was worried about leveraging my future; my response was not that I was worried about taking out a $50,000 business loan to get things started.

I simply said, "I don't know…" I'll never

forget John's response. He said, "Chance,

you will figure it out. That's what you do!"

At that moment I needed reassurance. I

needed someone to believe in me. John's

confidence in me had more of an impact

than he'll ever know.

In the course of the years from my

accidentally starting a Titans team to now,

there were so many moments about which I

reminisce and realize even the smallest

change of events might have made the

outcome of my journey very different. I guess that is the nature of all of our lives. Thank goodness for the many people like John Flading, Steve Vogel, Dennis Smith and Guerry Baldwin, each of whom played a vital part in my finding success.

Right before I resigned from East Cobb Baseball, I called my dad in North Carolina. We talked about the opportunity and excitement of starting my own business. He was excited for me, but also recognized the risk I was taking by leaving East Cobb. East Cobb had been where I had earned my stripes in the travel baseball world. It is where I earned the reputation of being a good coach. Venturing out on my own was exciting, but there was a lot of unknown.

When I talked to my dad, we went through the opportunity that had presented itself in regard to John Flading's facility that was somewhat ready for our transition. We talked about cost. We talked about the cost of the teams and attempted to identify what would motivate a parent to leave ECB in order to come with me to the newly minted

Titans Sports Academy. We made predictions about who would be loyal to the Titans and who would be loyal to ECB and why. What would be a deciding factor in these 120 families making the leap with me? What value proposition did the Titans offer that East Cobb did not or could not? What was my marketing plan? No one had ever tried to take on the proverbial 800 pound gorilla that was East Cobb Baseball and survived. What was the break-even point? How many teams did I need to make this work? What was the date that was the point of no return? Had I already passed that?

This sort of exodus from ECB was something no one had ever successfully navigated because no one wanted to test the might of the largest travel organization in the country; moreover no one had ever even attempted to pull away from East Cobb with more than one team and I was trying to do it with nine (nervous swallow.)

After much deliberation my father ended our phone call by making two points. The first scared me to death as it was a scenario I had not ever considered. My dad asked me,

"Chance you have thought long and hard about this. You have done your research and are prepared, but what happens if after you announce your plans to leave East Cobb and take all your Titans teams with you, Guerry finds nine coaches for your Titans and those coaches call the parents of players on those nine Titans teams and recruit them to stay at East Cobb. What if Guerry continues to call those teams East Cobb Titans? It would create enough chaos to potentially scatter many of the parents."

When I heard this, I immediately felt sick. I
had no answer for that scenario. My dad's
second point was this, "Chance, if you don't
do this you will regret it for the rest of your
life! You're ready!" And so on September
25, 2013, I turned in my resignation to East
Cobb Baseball, Inc. It was the last meeting I
had with Guerry Baldwin and it was a long
one.

I appreciate so many things Guerry did for
me for me during my decade at East Cobb. I
cherish my time there and know that the
Titan organization could never have become

what it is now, without that experience….

the good stuff and the bad.

Thursday, October 31, 2013

To: Guerry Baldwin President of East Cobb Baseball

East Cobb Baseball Board of Directors

East Cobb Baseball Staff

4617 Lee Waters Rd

Marietta, GA 30066

Mr. Baldwin, Board and Staff:

I wanted to write you personally to thank each of you for the roles you have played in my development and progression as a coach and individual over the past decade. In particular, I would like to thank Guerry Baldwin for his dedication to the East Cobb complex, his players and to the development of amateur baseball, as a whole. His friendship through this incredibly difficult decision of leaving East Cobb has been invaluable. Guerry has been a friend and mentor while also helping me both professionally and personally over my eleven years at East Cobb. Guerry's direction has helped me realize my dream of running a baseball organization, and I'm eternally grateful to him for that.

I would like to also thank the East Cobb Board of Directors for their support of the Academy during my time at East Cobb and the growth they have helped it to attain.

The Academy will be left in more than capable hands with Russ Dickerson and Ben Blumenthal as they will continue on with the Academy.

I would like to also the opportunity to thank Jeff Guy, Dennis Jordan, Wes Rynders, Dave Roberts and Juerod Roberts for their friendship and guidance with the Academy over the years. Folks like this are difficult to come by and I have appreciated their work and presence during my stay at ECB.

In closing, I am confident that I have helped East Cobb over the last 10+ Years and I'm proud of what we have accomplished during this time with not only the East Cobb Baseball Academy but also with the Titans organization. I wish East Cobb Baseball and each of you continued success in the future. I will continue to be an advocate of East Cobb even though I am moving on to focus on with Titans Sports Academy.

Once again, thank you all for your help and continued support.

Chance Beam, President

Titans Sports Academy

Inning #7 The Blue Print- The Foundation on Which Our Program Is Based

The creation and development of the Titans program is a lot like the construction of a tall building. A kcy factor in both is a structurally stable base or foundation. Accountability, responsibility, attitude, effort and integrity are the components of the foundation upon which our program has been built. I first embraced four of the five pillars that our program is based on in my Clemson Baseball Camp days many years ago. Back then Coach Wilhelm stressed that

accountability, responsibility, attitude and
effort would be needed and used all the days
of our lives.

Coach Wilhelm told a story about how if the
field needed to be raked, the typical player
would grab the rake and go about just raking
the area at home plate or first base. When
they got the job done well enough, they
would stop and put the rake away and go
about their business. But what if one of his
players or staff would look at that small task
as if it were something of value. As his
guys would give that task the proper attitude

and effort it deserved. As that player or staff member was accountable to his team for it being done and responsible for the task completion. Raking the field was just any task, it was only an opportunity to display accountability- I'm on this team and I want the best for them, Responsibility- I was tasked with raking the field, so it has to be done right, Attitude- The task was not to small, as no person is too big for any task and no project is too small, and lastly Effort- to give the proper energy to a task and see it to completion. At the end of the speech Coach Wilhelm said, "When you are done raking, you should be able and look and see that that is the best job of raking that has ever been done!" This story was a constant for Coach Wilhelm in the many years I attended camp. I bet I have told that story hundreds of time. The many coaches and/or players that had any interaction with Coach Wilhelm know that story well.

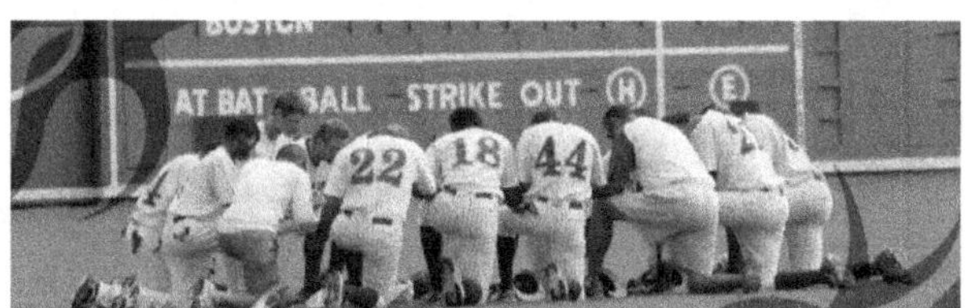

TEAM PRAYER BEFORE 2012 NATIONAL CHAMPIONSHIP GAME

In 2010, we had another good team. Two players in particular were very talented and were drawing a good bit of attention from colleges coaches. Sean McLaughlin, who eventually went to University of Georgia and was drafted in the nineteenth round by the Atlanta Braves and Nathan Mikolas, who was a third round pick by the New York Yankees out of high school in the 2012 MLB draft. We had a World Series in McKinney Texas for the AABC World Series. We had driven 12 hours down to the event from Atlanta. I got a call from a Randy Mazey, whom I had coached with at University of Tennessee in 2001 where we had taken a team to Omaha and finished third Nationally. Coach Mazey in 2010 was the recruiting coordinator at Texas Christian University (TCU). He asked me about my team and if McLaughlin and Mikolas were making the trip with my team to Texas. I assured him that they were. He asked if we had an afternoon off, if we could drive over to Fort Worth, that was about an hour away, so the guys could meet the Head Coach Jim Schlossnagle. I said yes. We played Saturday morning at 9 am and after we got back to the hotel I grabbed McLaughlin and Mikolas and we drove to Fort Worth.

Both Coach Randy Mazey and Coach Jim Schlossnagle were Clemson guys. Coach Mazey had played all four years at Clemson and was an assistant coach under Wilhelm

from 1990-1993. Coach Schlossnagle was

on the same staff under Coach Wilhelm in

1993, his last year as head coach of the

Tigers. To say these guys came from the

same coaching tree would be an

understatement.

When we got to Fort Worth that afternoon it

was approximately 4:00pm. I remember

that because as we walked in to the Stadium

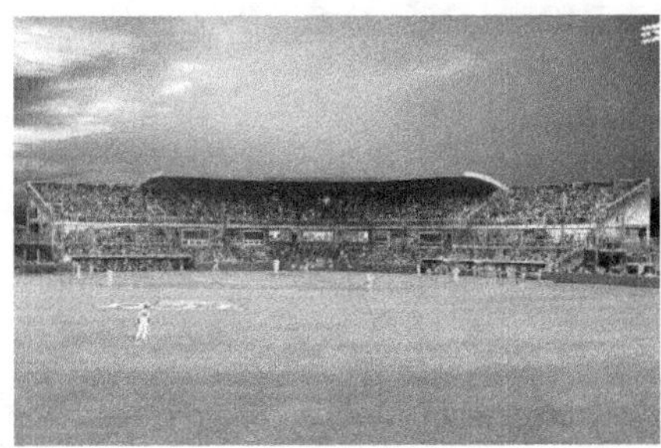 Coach

Schlossnagle

met us in the

third base dugout as about 150 high school players sat in the stands watching him give these two guys a personal tour of the facility. We toured the locker room and training facility. Meanwhile 150 other kids sat sweating in the Texas summer heat. I asked Schlossnagle who the kids in the stands were. He calmly mentioned they were there for a camp that started at 4:00pm, it was 4:25. We finished in Coach Schlossnagle office right behind home plate. As we walked into the office we noticed the office faced the field, it had floor to ceiling windows. It was a breath-taking view of an incredible facility. Coach Schlossnagle spoke with the guys briefly and told the

story about how their program was based on

accountability, responsibility, attitude and

effort. Coach Schlossnagle even told the

story about raking the dirt. As soon as we

walked out of the door of his office, both

players grabbed my arm, stopped me and

said, "Coach there is no way you didn't tell

him what to say there. He told the same

exact story you have told us countless

times." I laughed and explained we had all

grown from the coaching tree of Coach

Wilhelm. I went on to explain how we had

all heard that same speech countless times

and we all recited it to this day.

The values of accountability, responsibility, attitude, effort and integrity permeate every Titans practice and game. One may note that integrity was not in the four pillars Coach Wilhelm told. Integrity was added in 2014 as we found that it was the glue that holds the other pillars together. They are the pillars of our program and form the foundation of what we teach.

Our mission is to teach baseball and softball skills and to inspire hard work, winning attitudes, and respect for the "great and glorious game."* We hone outstanding sportsmen and women and fundamentally sound players capable of competing at the highest level that their maximum individual physical and mental capacities allow, whether on youth, high school, college, or professional diamonds. More importantly, in educating these developing young people in all facets of baseball and softball, we nurture the pattern of striving for excellence as they enter adulthood and become working professionals, servants in their communities, husbands, wives, fathers, mothers and the leaders who will sustain our future.

We believe that our time in practices and or games with our players is an opportunity to teach young people life skills. While we hope the fruits of our labor is seen on the field, it is far more important that we impact their lives. We build champions for the field and for life.

Players on my teams are expected to be accountable for their own equipment as well as all team equipment, including ball buckets. We don't assign specific players to specific pieces of equipment. If you see something which needs to be done, the expectation is that you do it. On one occasion, I got a call from a tournament director in Charleston, SC to let me know he had my team's ball bucket. I drove all the way back to the field to pick it up from him before heading back home to Georgia. There were 49 balls in that bucket. Realizing this was a teaching opportunity, once back in Marietta, I told the team they would not be allowed to practice until they earned back every single ball they had collectively left behind in South Carolina. One by one they did sets of 49 exercises. High Knees, push-up, lunges, crunches, and more to earn each and every ball back. They were accountable

for the balls, there was no upper class, no

underclass, just ownership of what belongs

to the team and that is not to be taken for

granted.

As a player you own your success. I have

never met a player who did not want to own

their success. I many times tell my teams

that success is only rented never owned. As

success is so fleeting. Baseball is a game of

failure. More times than not, it is through

failing that we learn our greatest lessons in

life. A great example of a player taking

personal responsibility, is a young man by the name of Ennis Coble. Ennis is one of my favorite players all time! He was not the fastest runner nor did he have the strongest arm, but he was a dynamic player because he took the responsibility of being a team player extremely seriously. Ennis, was highly intelligent. After I explained an expectation or rule to the team, Ennis would hang around after we broke the huddle and would say, "Hey coach, so when we hit a flyball to the outfield we have to run all the way to sprint all the way to second base no matter if the ball has been caught or not?" I would say, "Yes, Ennis on every flyball to the outfield you have to run all the way to second base." He would nod his head smile and then run off the do whatever he was to be doing next. It was like he was confirming the details and making certain he understood the expectation and then filed it away in his head almost as if he was inserting a home-made flash card into a box so he could pull it out and study it some more. He strove to execute every task to perfection every single time. He was the epitome of responsibility as he owned the task that he was given and executed them to an exacted standard.

Many of my players came to me as

underdogs. There are always very good

players who aren't quite good enough to

make the number one teams. We have

enjoyed tremendous success in the travel

baseball world by taking these players - the

ones who fell a little short on physical talent

- and teaching them how to become

producers by doing the little things right.

That starts with attitude. Often times

players who are short on size or strength or

speed or even some intangible quality

actually have a huge advantage over

physically more gifted athletes. With the

right attitude, short comings can become

great motivating factors. Playing with a

chip on one's shoulder – the intense desire

to prove oneself – is a recipe for the drive

and determination that makes the child in

your heart cry out, "I belong!" By

demanding our players embrace the attitude

of a champion, by setting high standards and

expectations, we help them enjoy success

that seems only reserved for the most

talented athletes

The attitude of a player drives his/ her

successes or failures. Our players have a

long list of *Chanceisms*, the list of one liners

I've assembled together over the years. The list is a long one, but the one that has stood the test of time is EVERYTHING MATTERS. Once, a number of years ago, I was sitting in the stands before the start of a game. EVERYTHING MATTERS was printed on the back of my t-shirt. A woman sitting in the stands close by read my shirt and commented to me that it must be stressful if "everything has to matter." I replied,

"Ma'am, if everything doesn't matter we need to find something else to do with our time." Everything matters is an attitude, not a chore. When

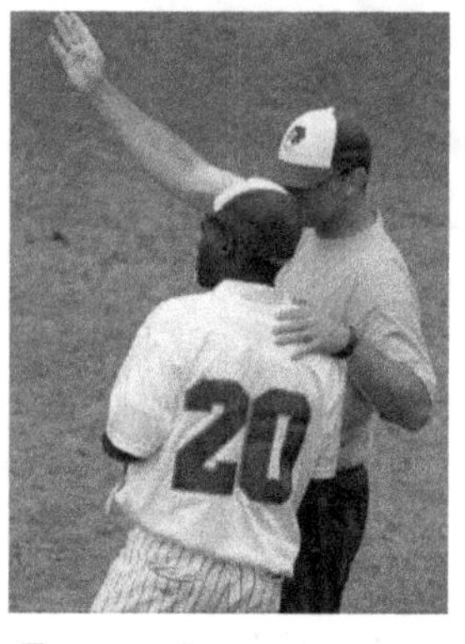

TALKING ANGLES WITH AN OUTFIELDER

everything matters you own your success and your failures. As a player when everything matters you are constantly engaged, not only in the physical, but also in the mental warfare of the game. Let's take focusing on the smallest detail or nuance of an opposing pitcher as he comes set as an example. You're a player on second base. The pitcher gets his sign from the catcher. You take your primary lead, which is done in an exact execution of walking steps - left, right, left… stay…you see the pitcher come set after receiving the signs, then you shuffle, shuffle and a half to max primary lead. You note that once the pitcher comes set he looks once, but he moves his head away and glances your way toward second base. He turns his head and pitches. Next pitch the pitcher comes set and does this again. The third pitch, the pitcher comes set he turns his heads to look at you at second base. The moment he moves his head back to look at home plate you break to third. The pitcher lifts his leg just as he has done in the previous two

pitches and doesn't notice that you have

broken to steal third base. You steal third

with no attempt from the catcher to make a

throw to third base. Did you steal third

because you're smarter than other players or

hustled more than the average player? No,

you stole third base because two innings

earlier you and your team noticed that the

pitcher was a one look guy when runners are

on second base. EVERYTHING

MATTERS because it puts players in a state

of constant cognitive engagement allowing

them to find the slightest edge and

exploiting that edge for the success of the

team. The game is won above the shoulders.

So is life.

Baseball in its essence is an easy sport. You

throw the ball, you hit the ball, and you

catch the ball. That's it. Effort is what's

done between all of that. Effort is what

makes the game go. Effort cannot be faked.

We have coached more than 700 players

who have gone on to play college or

professional baseball. Every single one of

those players were taught the importance of

effort. Effort is best described as giving your

physical effort when no one could be

watching.

A great example of effort comes with the

attitude that every defensive player on a

team has a job to do on every. When no

runners are on base and a ground ball is hit

to the left side of the field, the job of the

infielders not fielding the ball (including the

catcher) and the right fielder is to back up

the first basemen. They must be on or past

the foul line when the ball is caught at first

base. Many players take a few steps, see the

play is going to be made and simply stop.

They sell themselves and their team short

with a lack of effort on the one play. Later

in the game the same play happens the same

defense men make very little effort to back

up first base on the ground ball. The third

baseman makes a hard throw to the first

baseman it sails past his glove, bouncing off

the fence behind first base and shooting

down the right field line in foul territory.

The right fielder, now realizing he did not

give full effort must spring toward the ball

as it careens down the right field line. The

base runner sees the ball sail over the first

baseman's head and immediately turns on

the jets to get to get to second base. The

baserunner glides in to second base with no throw. Next hitter hits a ground ball to second base to move the runner to third base to record one out. The next hitter hits a long fly ball in which the runner tags up and scores from third base. The team is down 1-0. The team loses 1-0. Was the play lost on the lack of one hustle play? No… Their many at bats and plays that could have changed the entire game, but what if the right fielder had of backed up the base every time and gave great effort. What would have the score been?

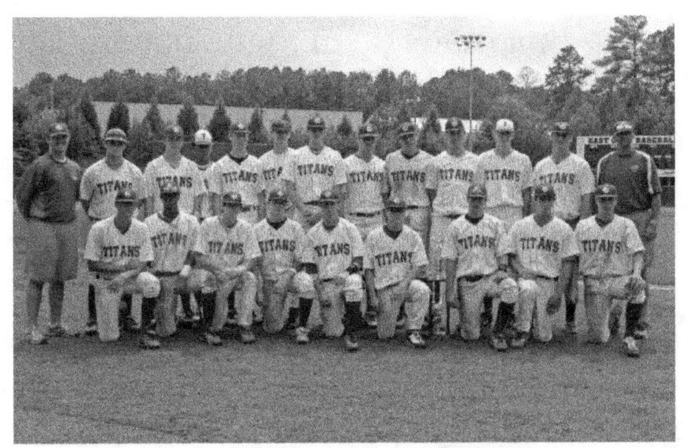
2009 AABC National Champions

I often joke that Jesus was high on integrity.
Integrity within the Titans program is taught
through our other principles of
responsibility, accountability, effort and
attitude. Integrity is doing the right thing
even when no one is watching. In many
ways, integrity is the glue that binds it all
together. Having a great attitude and
hustling is all fine and good, but it's

integrity that binds them to the betterment of

the teams. A player can be accountable for

his actions, but the integrity is what allows

him to hold his head high when he is done

playing because he knows there is nothing

he left undone. Integrity is what allows a

player to have no regrets when the game is

done.

We believe that our time in practices and

games with our players is an opportunity to

teach young people life skills. While we

hope the fruits of our labor is seen on the

field, it is far more important that we impact

their lives. Accountability, responsibility, attitude, effort and integrity is the foundation of Titans Sports Academy. We build champions in baseball and softball, but most important we build champions for life.

POST GAME

In a world where everything seems so random, old principles still work. I had a vision in the Spring of 2008 about a thing that, at that point, I didn't know how to describe. I dreamt of blue walls and slogan scattered throughout our facility. I dreamt of a parent waiting rooms with closed caption TV's. I dreamed that we would someday have our very own field.

Our core principle works of Accountability, Responsibility, Attitude, Effort, and

Integrity worked 20 years ago and they will

work 20 years from now. I truly believe that

while the Titans have been blessed beyond

comprehension, our success all boils down

to the 5 pillars that we layout in this book. I

am not the smartest guy. Writing this book

has been like fingernails being screeched

down a chalkboard, but in the consummate

fashion of all things in which I have thrown

myself and suffered through this process

relying on these core principles.

I believe that our core principles of

accountability, responsibility, attitude,

effort, and integrity shape young players and their game daily. More importantly, I believe that these principles will shape the next sixty years of life. Accountability, responsibility, attitude, effort, and integrity are often difficult to embody, but these attributes are time tested. Living a life well lived never goes out of style and always succeeds!

Why Are We Titans? By: Jason Fincher

My son began playing for the Titans at the age of 9, he is now 15. So, needless to say, we have been around for a while. In fact, we are what I would refer to as "repeat Titans." My son left to play for another organization at the age of 12, and came back to the Titans the year after and has been there ever since. Having been with another organization and then returning, we can honestly say there's nowhere else we would want our son to play.

There are many reasons why we chose the

Titans initially and then chose to return.

The single biggest

reason why we love

the Titans is simple.

They genuinely care

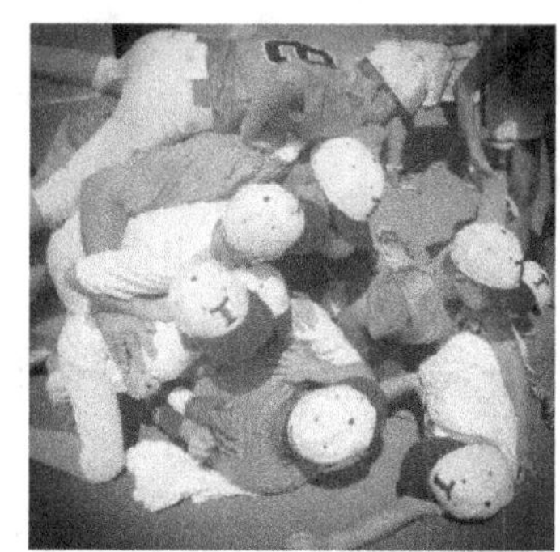

about their players. Sure, they care about

whether or not your child succeeds on the

baseball field, but with the Titans it is so

much bigger than that. Chance and his staff

genuinely care about not only developing

baseball players, but developing young men

who will become great husbands, fathers,

and leaders in the community.

For two years now, my son has had the privilege of having Chance Beam as his head coach. My family and I have been around travel baseball for a very long time, I myself had the privilege of playing travel and college baseball as a young man and I have seen and played for countless coaches over the years. There is nobody that we would rather play for and be associated with than the Titans.

This past weekend, we played in a Memorial Day baseball tournament and ended up having to play 2 games on Memorial Day.

The team played extremely well and ended

up winning the championship, going 6-0 on

the weekend, but it's what happened prior to

our first game on Memorial Day that

summarizes why we chose the Titans. We

arrived at the park at 7AM for an 8AM

game, as I walked into the park I noticed the

team was huddled around Coach Beam at

the batting cage, but nobody was warming

up at the time. As I got closer, I overheard

Coach Beam reminding the players that it

was Memorial Day and what that means and

why they even get the opportunity to play

baseball in the first place. Life lessons,

that's truly what all this is about, and

Chance and his staff are second to none.

We left the Titans a few years ago because

we thought the "grass was greener on the

other side." We quickly found out that was

not the case and that we had made a mistake.

Not once during that year did we feel like

our son was cared for like he was during his

time with the Titans. When the time came

to pick a team for the following year, the

decision was easy, we were returning to the

Titans.

Accountability, responsibility, and integrity are three core principles the Titans believe in. They just don't say it, they live it. The players with the Titans are held accountable, and are required to be responsible young men of the highest character. It is truly evident that developing baseball players is not their sole mission. Sure, it is an important one and why we invest so much time and money in the game, but deep down we all know that baseball will come to an end and these players need to be equipped to be good men, husbands, fathers and citizens. That, in a nutshell, is why we are Titans and always will be.

The Notebook by: Mike Nayman

The Fine Line Between Success and Failure Chronicled in a Spiral Notebook

This portion of the Titans history needs a bit of background. My relationship with Chance Beam started in September of 2011 with a phone call I took in the parking lot of the Disney All-Star resort in Orlando. I was on a family vacation and received a call inquiring about possibly coaching for the Titans in the summer of 2012. I had never spoken to Chance before, that phone call, but two hours later, I had a new coaching gig and an upset family. Never before had an 80-degree Florida evening felt so cold. My wife and kids totally froze me out for about 24 hours. Bad mistake on my part (or so I thought at the time), but either way, my sojourn into travel baseball had begun. I had no idea what to expect nor did I have an idea of what was to come or how it would impact my outlook on the game that I loved. As it turned out, I found new ways not only to coach, but also new ways to deal with players and parents. I also learned that baseball is business even for young players, especially working toward playing at the next level. It opened my eyes to many things with the realization that it's not always about winning games.

Can You Handle the Truth?

Sometimes the difference between brilliance and foolishness, good and bad or right and wrong is all in the eyes of the beholder. To think things are so clear cut that any rational person can tell the difference isn't always the case. Early in on in Titans history, trying to determine success from failure simply wasn't possible. With no true baseline to measure what would bring a plan to fruition, often times it was like shooting in the dark.

Basically when Chance asked me my opinion on things, I simply shot straight and gave him the answer that I thought was best. That certainly didn't mean it was correct nor was it always what he wanted to hear. I spoke in terms of what I thought would be most effective or what would bring the biggest success. I gave opinions without considering any consequences should my ideas render failure or whether it was what Chance wanted to hear. I was honest and forthcoming.

The true beauty of my relationship with the Titans was more in the context of a counterbalance. It was my feeling that if Chance was going to lean on me, I always had to be honest with my answers and open with my thoughts. Ironically, I think a portion of the Titans organization is built upon this foundation. It has never been the mantra of the organization to sugar-coat an observation or an evaluation. Just to be clear, it is also against the organization's belief system to tear down the dreams or goals of a youngster. Simply put, be honest and lend a helping hand when possible. While there are always extenuating circumstances, I am proud to have been associated with the Titans all these years. I would rather keep honesty a top priority rather than raising false hope throughout the ranks.

Big Hat and No Cattle

Fake it 'til you make it might be the most artful way to describe my method of dealing with Chance and his visions. I became a walking think tank for the organization. I often joke with Chance that any time he asks for my opinion, it's going to cost him money! I would come up with the ideas, he would come up with the checks. It really was a great relationship from my point of view. If I imagined it, Chance found a way to breathe life into the idea. It would soon have a heartbeat – a pulse that might be weak or one that was seemingly filled with adrenaline. We could pull the plug at any time or we may transform it into a monster that Dr. Frankenstein would be proud to call his own. Believe me when I say that we dabbled at both ends of this spectrum.

Nothing seemed too big, nor too small. From large murals on the wall to the smallest of logos on a piece of paper. If an idea popped into my head, we discussed bringing it to fruition. This method was truly one of the hidden gems of the Titans while also being one of the genuine joys of my friendship with Chance Beam.

Nothing is out of bounds and nothing ever seems too grand or too insignificant to consider. I think it's the open-mindedness that has guided the Titans organization to its current success.

What made this a unique way of doing business, is that most of these ideas required a lot of time, effort, people, players, equipment, teams, knowledge, permits, plans, drawings, architects, bank loans, space, facilities, travel and, of course, money.

Everything sounded great and was good on paper, but at some point, rubber had to meet pavement and we had to have *cattle*. The Titans looked the part and acted the part. In fact, we played the part on the field. The Titans have always been competitive when it came to playing the game. While I have my own theories on the actual success of our teams, I will leave that for another author and chapter.

We needed cattle, lots and a lots of it. The obvious question, "How do we grow the business?"

Don't' Dwell on What You Don't Have. Dream About What You Will Go Out and Get

We never seemed to spend much time worrying about what other programs had in terms of championships or 5-star players. If we followed our game plan, it would surely bring long-term success. There was that fine line again… the one that was omnipresent at every turn.

The reality for us back in the early 2010's was that many people actively involved in the organization were not a part of the grassroots travel ball program that Chance took a shot in starting when he left East Cobb. In fact, I never even saw those days. I jumped in just as Chance and the Titans were hitting second gear.

The difference between those days and where we are today is like night and day. In 2019, it is open throttle on a long, flat highway. The speed limit is irrelevant. However, the one thing that the organization has never done is put it on cruise control. We seemed to always be accelerating with the thought that a cruising speed was viewed as complacency – which is the first sign of demise.

So where, exactly, did this methodology of projected growth come from?

Old School Methods Produce New School Practicality

Chance's initial vision aside, the methods we employ in running the organization today started in a hotel room in Florida. A seismic event took place and we didn't even know it happened. The process was simple and primitive. The results started a domino effect that could only be described as interesting. And to think it all started with a notebook and a pen, not a laptop, tablet or even smartphone, is unfathomable in this day and age, but that's precisely how things got started.

It was commonplace for us to travel to tournaments together via truck or plane. Usually Chance would drive, I would talk for long periods of time, he would listen and we'd swap roles along the way. It would not only pass the time, but often times we'd strike oil. Looking back on these numerous road trips, it was almost disappointing if we didn't come up with the next great idea by the time we returned home.

Chance and I would often sit and talk and throw out some of the craziest ideas regarding baseball, business and life in a totally random thought process. Often times, we missed the boat, so to speak. We'd percolate an idea that seemed great, but inevitably we would forget some of our best material by the time we

reconvened back in Marietta. We never wrote stuff
down. I guess we just thought we would remember
everything we thought of during our most recent trip.

Age certainly plays tricks on the mind. We lost many
details and revolutionary thoughts on how to change
baseball as those mile markers ticked by the various
southern states through which we traveled. The details
are a bit fuzzy, but I definitely claim credit for the best
Titans idea ever, which was investing $1.99 in an actual
notebook. It was nothing fancy, just your garden variety
spiral-bound, real paper notebook. With that first
notebook we became officially official! No more lost
ideas. No more forget the details. We meant business.

This notebook would go on to contain the most secret of innovations to the world of travel baseball. If it were to fall into enemy hands it would surely mean doom and destruction to the Titans empire!

While that certainly sounds like a great movie trailer, the reality was that it proved to be a consistent way for us to record ideas, to kick the tires on some topics or simply have a framework in place that we could revisit at a later time.

It has long been my opinion that if the casual observer were to duck into a conversation midstream with Chance and me, not only would they not be able to understand what we were talking about, but they also would be curious as to how we even arrived on the topic.

In an odd way, Chance and I probably speak our own language. Often times, we may have a we may not speak for weeks, but when we reconnect it seems like we're picking up right where we left off without skipping a beat. Random thoughts, random texts and outlandish conversations are an integral part of our working relationship and our friendship

Anyway, while I will take full credit for the notebook (whether that is fact or fiction, it's not relevant at this point – it just makes for a better story), I may have even suggested to Chance that he use the 'notes app' on his phone. That way, when a random idea popped up that seemed too good or big to be true, he was covered. Jot it down!!!

The Proof is in the Pudding

While this modus operandi may have seemed liked an exercise in futility, only time would tell. When we would re-visit these thoughts or how we would take action on them had no bearing on the random and often times impulsively scribbled notes. Ultimately, it provided a safe place to store your imagination so that more thoughts, definition or dimension could be added in the future. It was like having a memory stick for your laptop – we just weren't that technical at the time.

We literally started writing down things that we wanted to see take place for the Titans. A virtual crystal ball full of wishes, dreams and prognostications. When a new thought popped up, we would just add another number to the growing list of possibilities. That notebook that Chance carried became the mobile think-tank for the shape and future of the Titans organization. If something made it in to that spiral bound, paper pack, it was in play. No questions asked. No filters. It was now in play.

As we have looked back at this keepsake over the years, some of the ideas were absolutely lead balloons. Not only were they never getting off the ground, but they would become areas that bogged us down if we allowed ourselves to spend too much time with them. However, one of the most subtle lessons learned was that no idea was a bad idea. They were all vetted equally and some simply didn't make the cut for whatever reason. This very process was another one of the foundational principles that continues to shape the Titans today.

Regardless, failure was never feared. Even bad ideas kept the imagination flowing. Looking back, I guess this led to the reasoning process that would only lead us to other great ideas in the future. If a garden was truly going to grow, seeds would have to be planted and unconditional care would have to be given with no results guaranteed.

While none of our ideas were ever sure things, the amazing part about our process was that more times than not, most of the ideas proved to be positive experiences. They would lead us into broader areas and directions that would eventually catapult the organization. Goals were set financially and physically, which led directly to the plan of eventual facilities that would rival any in the industry. This seed was planted in that inaugural notebook during our first Florida hotel room brainstorming scribble-fest. We just started writing down everything that came to mind over the course of a couple of hours on that trip and as crazy as it sounds, some of the best, long-lasting goals and methods for achieving them in Titans history were given life on this trip. The notebook proves it!

We often questioned ourselves on matters of the

number of teams, age groups, coaches, equipment and

staffing that would be needed in order to take the next

leaps forward. How could a facility be modernized and

accommodate all of the needs of the organization?

What would be the ideal price points and profit margins

for these ventures? What was the ceiling that could be

achieved in gross income and where might the net

profit settle in? One thing Chance has never shied away

from is the fact that at the end of the day, if the Titans

organization is going to provide the best instruction and

functionality in the travel baseball world, it ALSO has

to be treated as a business.

Even an Old Dog Can Learn New Tricks

Of all the things I would say to Chance over the years in jest, in seriousness, in frustration or for any reason, the one word never uttered between us was *softball.* Whether it was by calculated avoidance or it simply never came up in conversation, we never contemplated adding softball to our menu of services. The irony of this in both of our lives could never be fully explained to the point of giving it justice. As baseball men through and through, the grand ole game would always be king and there was no room in the discussion for anything else, but fate has a sense of humor. My wife, Kendra, and I were blessed with a daughter and a son. Neither of which had any true interest in the sport of baseball. They tolerated it, dabbled in it during their youth, but ultimately found other sports and interests as they grew older. Chance and his wife, Christine, were blessed with two lovely girls that followed along much the same path as my own children. Baseball was a part of their lives, but it did not consume them the way it did their father. Between us, few had for our children and two wives who tolerated the game, but didn't revere it in the same way Chance and I did. And here is where the plot thickens.

I took on the additional role as head softball coach at Creekview High School to go along with my head baseball coaching position at the school. It would eventually culminate in Creekview winning a Georgia state softball title and a genuine love and appreciation for softball. Around the same time, Chance's oldest daughter, Brooke, was developing into a top-flight fastpitch softball youth pitcher with an extremely bright future. Suddenly softball, which neither of us ever considered bringing into the Titan's organization, became a hot topic.

I am not sure when or how it happened, but I remember suggesting we should look at developing softball within the Titans' footprint. If we could go back to a point earlier in this chapter when we highlighted the point that EVERY idea received equal consideration. Well, that may have been a bit of wishful thinking. I think the conversation was as simple as "Hey, Chance. Have you ever thought about adding…*softball*?" There it was. I said it with optimal fervor. "Softball." Silence. Crickets. A stare. What had I done?

Softball? Why not?! It ended up being one of the transformational changes in the Titans organization. It broadened the horizons and was one more idea brought to fruition that contributed to the evolution of the Titans. Softball brought a monumental change to the business that proved to expand the limits of where the Titans' ceiling. A glass ceiling, so to speak, that would be smashed in the very near future.

In addition to softball, major changes in philosophy, facilities, branding, corporate partners and sponsorships were all being addresses. How and where would we acquire players for the future? Who was our competition? Where was the point of satisfaction in all of this? Can we ever be too big for our own good?

There were many unknowns, but we were never scared to walk into and out of the dark. Fear was never a factor. at least for me. I had no fiscal responsibility in the operation. I was just a camp instructor, a coach, a sounding board and an idea guy. My skin in the game was never in danger of being scraped away. That responsibility fell totally on Chance.

At the end of the day, when looking back at it, Chance and I absolutely needed to be two separate entities. If my thoughts were limited based on financial responsibility or a biased point of view, I'm not sure some of the ideas I threw at him would've ever come

full circle. On the flipside, if Chance ever said we need

to limit what could be spent or how we could spend it, I

think that may have also put limitations on what he

would consider for the future of the organization.

Ultimately, the boundaries, or lack there-of, really

allowed for the growth of the organization. I think

Chance knew it would take money in order to make

money and because of this, the idea of a million-dollar

complex never seemed out of reach to him. In fact, as

time went on, it not only became an achievable reality,

but it also proved to be a necessity. Through the

consistent growth of the program in terms of scope,

teams, players and necessity, a large indoor structure as

well as an outdoor field were needed if the Titans were going to reach its potential.

As I reflect on the ideas, both foolish and brilliant, contained within that spiral bound notebook, it reminds me of a genie's lamp. If we rubbed it just right and made a wish, often times our wishes would materialize. Little did we know at the time that this magic notebook was becoming the roadmap to where the organization has landed today at 775 Hawkins Store Road, Northeast, in a city in Georgia called Kennesaw.

Pictures from over the years

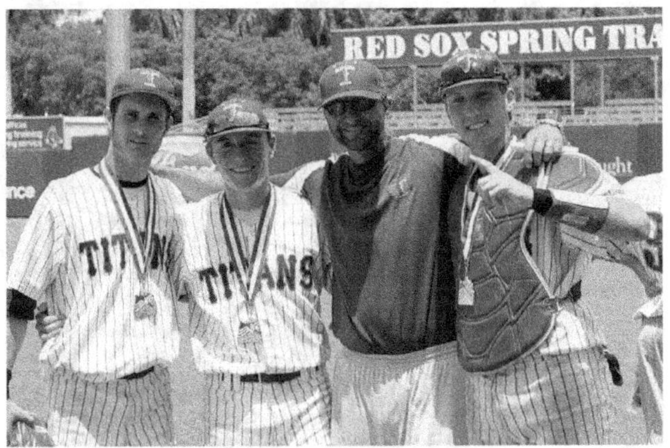

2010 AAU WORLD SERIES

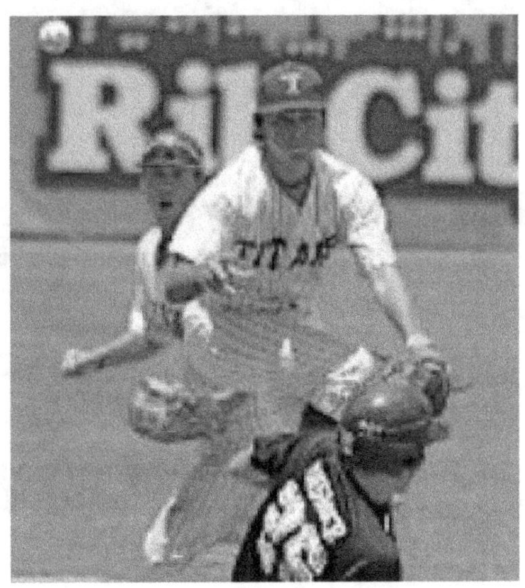

LAST PLAY OF 2010 AAU WORLD SERIES

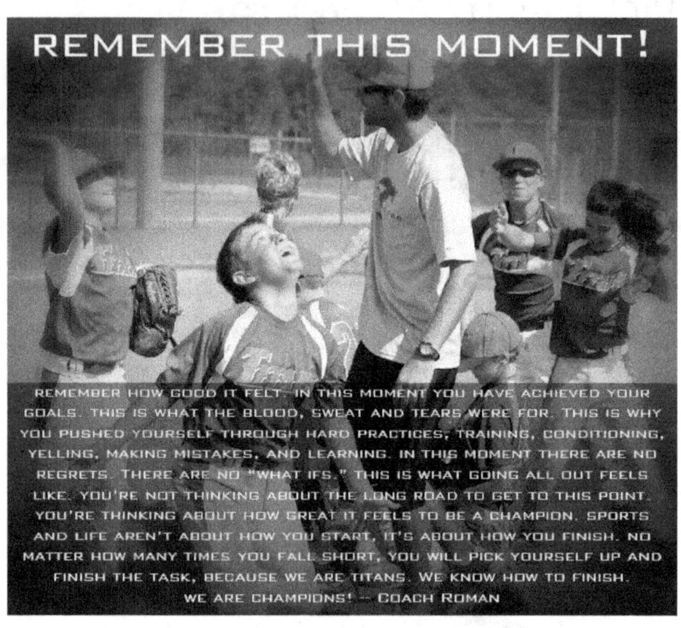

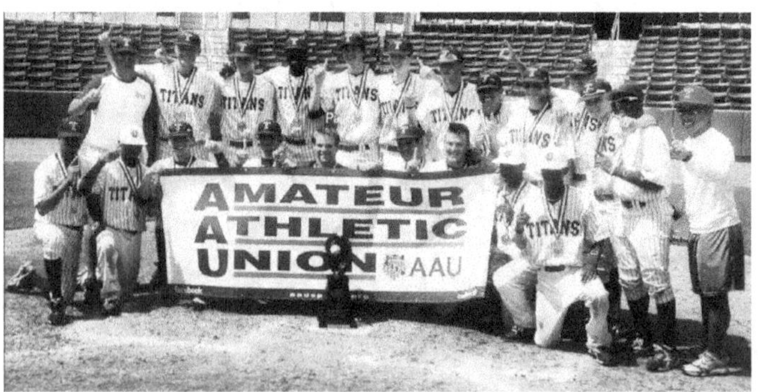

2012 AAU National Champions

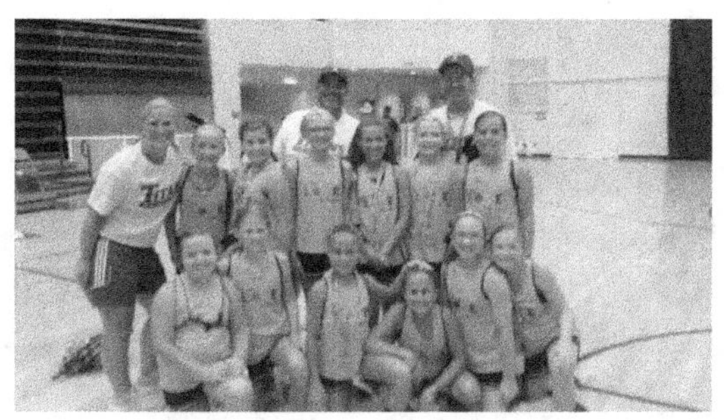

First Titans Fastpitch 2015

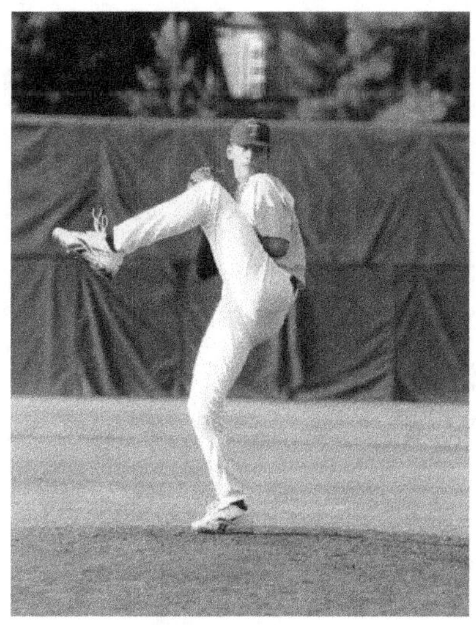

Nathaniel Lowe 1 of 5 to MLD Debut 2019

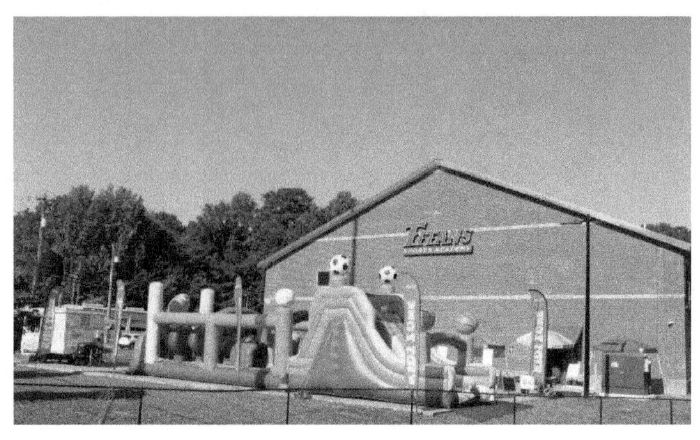

GRAND OPENING AT HAWKINS STORE RD - 2017